MANAGING TO NURSE:
INSIDE CANADA'S HEALTH CARE REFORM

How does the restructuring of health care in Canada affect nursing practice? Increasingly since the 1970s, and especially under recent reforms, a new style of information-supported, professionally based management has been implemented in Canadian health care. In *Managing to Nurse*, Janet M. Rankin and Marie L. Campbell probe the operation of this new managerialism in the hospital setting and its effect on nurses and nursing practice.

Written from a nursing perspective, this institutional ethnography documents a major transformation in the nature of nursing and associated patient care, and demonstrates how this work is now organized according to an 'accounting logic,' in which a cost orientation is embedded into care-related activities. Rankin and Campbell illustrate how nurses adapt to – and perpetuate – this system and how they learn to recognize their adaptations as professionally correct and as an adequate basis for professional judgement and practice. In addressing contemporary approaches to health care reform, *Managing to Nurse* provides an insiders' account that offers convincing evidence that nurses' caring work and patient welfare are being undermined, sometimes dangerously, by current health care agendas.

JANET M. RANKIN is a professor of nursing in the Faculty of Health and Human Services at Malaspina University-College.

MARIE L. CAMPBELL is a professor emerita in the Faculty of Human and Social Development at the University of Victoria.

JANET M. RANKIN AND MARIE L. CAMPBELL

Managing to Nurse
Inside Canada's Health Care Reform

UNIVERSITY OF TORONTO PRESS
Toronto Buffalo London

© University of Toronto Press Incorporated 2006
Toronto Buffalo London
Printed in Canada

ISBN-13: 978-0-8020-8013-4 (cloth)
ISBN-10: 0-8020-8013-8 (cloth)

ISBN-13: 978-0-8020-3791-6 (paper)
ISBN-10: 0-8020-3791-7 (paper)

Printed on acid-free paper

Library and Archives Canada Cataloguing in Publication

Rankin, Janet M. (Janet Mary), 1956–
    Managing to nurse : inside Canada's health care reform / Janet M.
Rankin and Marie L. Campbell.

    Includes bibliographical references and index.
    ISBN-13: 978-0-8020-8013-4 (bound)
    ISBN-10: 0-8020-8013-8 (bound)
    ISBN-13: 978-0-8020-3791-6 (pbk.)
    ISBN-10: 0-8020-3791-7 (pbk.)

    1. Nursing services – Canada – Administration.   2. Nursing – Canada.
3. Health care reform – Canada.   I. Rankin, Janet M.   II. Campbell,
Marie L. (Marie Louise), 1936–   III. Title.

RT89.R35 2006   362.17′3′068   C2005-905921-4

This book has been published with the help of a grant from the Canadian
Federation for the Humanities and Social Sciences, through the Aid to
Scholarly Publications Programme, using funds provided by the
Social Sciences and Humanities Research Council of Canada.

University of Toronto Press acknowledges the financial assistance to
its publishing program of the Canada Council for the Arts and the
Ontario Arts Council.

University of Toronto Press acknowledges the financial support for its
publishing activities of the Government of Canada through the
Book Publishing Industry Development Program (BPIDP).

To our teachers and students,
from whom we continue to learn.

Contents

Figures

MANAGING TO NURSE

Introduction

A Nursing Day Begins

It is 7:30 a.m., and outside the hospital, the sky is still dark. Nurses arrive at hospital wards for the day shift, most of them wearing pastel pantsuits and athletic shoes. Each wears a name tag that identifies her or his status as Registered Nurse or Licensed Practical Nurse. On Ward A the day nurses gather at the Nursing Station, check a printout of assignments posted on the wall, pick up paper and pencils, and go into the meeting room behind the desk. Listening to a tape-recorded message, they are getting the 'shift-change report.' One floor below, on Ward B, the change-over routine is slightly different. The newly arrived nurses check a written report left by the night staff, a tick-sheet that summarizes the night-time condition of their patients – their sleep, pain, confusion, incontinence, IV management, and so on – and they make notes, before heading out to begin their work with patients. This is the way an ordinary day begins for these nurses who are taking up their routine tasks as proficient members of a health care team.

This book problematizes the apparent routineness of nurses' work. As health care is being transformed in response to a variety of acute challenges, the question arises about how nurses are experiencing that transformation. More and more, a 'typical' shift of duty is fraught with changing demands and new complexities (Armstrong et al., 1994, 2000). Not that much attention is paid to what nurses do! The special skills and knowledge that nurses bring to health care are much more likely to be noted in their absence than celebrated in their accomplishment. One common complaint from hospital authorities is about what they see as the lack of readiness for work of new nurse graduates

(Utley-Smith 2004). Addressing schools of nursing, especially when a curriculum changes, hospitals anxiously demand that newly qualified nurses have adequate practical experience to step in and immediately do the job. For some time, it has been noted that a gap exists between the classroom and the workplace that nurses themselves must fill (Kramer 1974; 1981). Nursing educators recognize it as what they call a widening 'theory–practice gap.'[1] But we are not content to treat it as 'lack of practical experience' or misapplication of nursing theory. It appears to be dynamic, not static, and it affects all nurses, not just new graduates. Older, experienced nurses are also criticized for hanging on to outmoded ideas and, when they don't adapt, for being rigid, slow workers, or even 'burned out.'[2] The problems for nurses are variously conceptualized but are usually understood as something nurses themselves or nursing education should fix.

Although complaints about new nurses' readiness for work and experienced nurses' incapacities may have some basis in actuality, this book takes a different tack in conceptualizing and exploring them. As sociologists as well as nurses, we are interested in the social setting of nurses' work, and this chapter introduces that conceptualization.

We have been impressed by certain rather taken-for-granted features of nurses' work; for the practice of contemporary health care to proceed smoothly, or at all, nurses must and do produce and maintain the necessary terrain – a project that is always background, never foreground in accounts of their work. Nurses' work in hospitals holds a clinical environment together, making it run smoothly, creating it as a space where health caring activity can proceed. As health care reform is bringing new ideas to bear on the organization of hospitals, we wonder how nurses contribute to or are affected by what is happening. This book presents research that identifies and analyses some of the important transformations that have been occurring over several decades in Canadian hospitals. In what follows, we treat nurses doing their 'routine' jobs as experts in what they do; and our research proceeds by learning from them not just what they do but how they know to do it. It begins where nurses are and with their everyday experiences.

The authors, Janet Rankin and Marie Campbell, are researchers who, prior to becoming academics, both worked as nurses. Rankin is currently an instructor in an undergraduate nursing program. Campbell recently retired from a university faculty position where she taught nurses, among graduate students from other human service professions, and supervised their graduate research. When Rankin and

Campbell conduct participant observations in hospital settings, they recognize both continuity and change in how nurses work. Their ethnography provides the experiential basis for analysing just such features of the social organization. Examining the notes Rankin has taken during participant observation at the beginning of a day's work in 2004, we can see that these nurses get daily workload assignments in much the same way as nurses did in 1959 and 1979, when Campbell and Rankin, respectively, were working as nurses. Although nowadays the assignment sheet is computer-generated, it still lists the beds on the ward by room number and assigns nurses to patients accordingly. On this particular shift, Registered Nurse Linda McIvor, with her assistant, Licensed Practical Nurse Sara Green, will be responsible for the patients in rooms numbered from 235 to 238; these patients are recovering from surgery. Since two of the rooms are four-bedded, and two are doubles, this means that together Nurse Linda and Nurse Sara will be caring for twelve post-surgical patients.

At the meeting featuring a recorded shift-change report, some things look similar, and some rather different, from meetings of this sort forty-five or twenty-five years previously. Nurses dress differently than Campbell did in 1959, no longer in starched caps, bibs, and aprons. The pressed white scrub dresses that Rankin's generation of nurses wore in 1979 are gone as well. The interaction among the nurses is different, too. No longer is a night nurse responsible to stay and verbally report her 'hand-over' to the oncoming staff. Occasionally, a night nurse will delay her departure to speak privately to the nurse taking over from her, if she is anxious about something in her patients' care. But instead of the routine hand-over, with night nurses being there to tell the day nurses what happened during the night, the report will now be audio-taped or simply written. In 1959, and still in 1979, the Head Nurse for the ward would have been the central figure at a shift-change. The other nurses would have gathered around her and faced her. After listening to the night-nurse's report, she would have reviewed with her staff the individual nursing plans for the day of patient care. The plans would have been noted in a paper file called a Kardex and updated in pencil during the shift-change meeting (and as needed during the day). Held in this format, transcribed from doctors' orders and other sources, and available at the desk for nurses to consult was the patient-specific information that nurses needed in order to care for individual patients. No Head Nurse is present today at the shift-change meeting. Rather, one of the Registered Nurses coming on shift has been assigned, besides a workload of patients, the additional responsibility for being 'in charge' of all the patients and the care nurses will give that day.

Rankin's observations of shift-change caught nurses reviewing plans, sometimes discussing them briefly, and making notes on their daily worksheets, just as nurses would have done in earlier times. The same air of efficiency and briskness was observed. But new language and different issues now permeate the nurses' talk. Today, for instance, Sara, the Licensed Practical Nurse, mentions that one of her patients, elderly Mrs Light, should be made ALC. This designation of ALC is puzzling to us. It is not a medical diagnosis that we recognize, and indeed, were we to look, it would not be found in any official classification of diseases. But at the shift-change meeting, if seems that the other nurses are familiar with the term and that they agree with Sara's judgement. Another new topic features in the morning interchange between the nurse in charge and the day staff: the charge nurse consults a computer-generated list and announces how many beds are required for incoming patients that day. She approaches individual nurses as they leave the nursing station to begin their work, inquiring as to where their assigned patients are on their clinical pathways and whether their discharge plans are complete.

Not recognizing some of the language used at this shift-change, or at least the significance of what was said, we have to assume that we researchers fail to grasp everything that was going on. But nevertheless we think that we can see some things that are being accomplished. The nurses are getting instructions for their day's work, not all of them explicit, of course. That is, within the report and subsequent quick discussions, we do not see or hear detailed nursing instructions being given. Nurses are not sharing nursing 'tips.' Rather, they seem to be accumulating certain crucial bits of information about their assigned patients and the day's already scheduled plans for them. We assume that the nurses' undertakings are being coordinated within a complex of diagnostic and therapeutic actions and organizational processes of which nursing is only one part. We recognize that the nurses are bringing to bear their own sources of knowledge on the outlined plans. They are expected to know what to do, given this scaffolding of the day's work. As already noted, we hear references being made to activities whose specific content and meaning remain unexplained. Some of those references seem to be in 'codes' such as 'ALC' and 'Clinical Pathways.' While the notion of 'discharge' is commonplace, its prominence in the charge nurse's talk is new and puzzling. We see that the nurses themselves respond to the shift-change report with its more or less explicit, and more or less coded, instructions by making their own written notes and pocketing them. These notes, we expect from our own historical experience, will aid their memory all day about key points of intervention, scheduled deadlines, and elements of routine nursing care. In summary, we see nurses who are already knowledge-able caregivers interacting with and making use of organized and authoritative systems of knowing that are meant to guide and support both therapeutic and organizational action.

Knowledge for Taking Action

Our analysis in this book focuses on the intersection of different kinds of knowledge – of the caregivers' own knowing being brought together with other, externally derived and explicitly organized, systems of information.[3] The cursory examination we have just given to some observations of a shift-change report offers a tiny glimpse into certain routine aspects of nurses' work. For our purposes, it suggests that, over time, different *forms of knowledge* may become a coordinating feature of what nurses do. In this book we identify and analyse what some people see as a major transformation in how hospitals manage their internal operations, including the work of professionals. The word 'restructuring' is often applied to such organized transformation. Because these systematic transformations are fuelled by explicit and specialized information, *knowledge for taking action* in health care has moved into a position of primary importance.

At first glance, it may appear, simply, that as health care technology and hospital systems change, nurses' knowledge of how to participate has had to keep up. It is certainly the case that for the past forty years or so, nursing educators, researchers, and theorists, as well as the repre-sentatives of nursing's professional bodies have been compiling and using nursing knowledge to carve out and support nurses' unique con-tribution to health care. In that time nursing has become an academic discipline with a strong and growing research base. Curricula grounded in nursing scholarship have replaced the earlier 'training' of new nurses through apprenticeship types of education.[4] Adaptations in nurses' professional practice are also being accomplished within an ongoing transformation of health administration. Nurses join an extended dialogue among all the stakeholders in Canadian health care

– politicians, public sector policymakers and administrators, academic researchers and consultants, the health professions, and even citizens – that draws attention to a need to reform the health care system. A certain consensus has emerged that health care should be managed more efficiently, a direction that affects caregiving. No longer is it sufficient for caregivers to ask, 'What is it I need to know and do to help my patient?' Now nurses must know what they can do for their patients that brings the best value for money spent. Nor is this new formulation of nursing responsibility left up to individual caregivers to interpret as they see fit. As we argue in Chapter 1, health care reform makes it a systematic undertaking. Hospitals are being restructured to reap the benefits of more systematized and rationally managed delivery of health services. One focus of our analysis is the divergence that appears between the concept of nursing that nurses learn in their professional education and what they meet in everyday practice settings.

Transformations in Health Care

Reform is going forward in many health care settings, under many guises and interpretations, in various programs and activities, originating inside the health professions and external to them. An approach to managing called the new public management appears to be part of the restructuring efforts in Canada's public sector. McCoy (1998) reports that central to organizational restructuring is the work of 'making visible' and knowable whatever is to be managed. In this regard, the new public management brings a specific set of knowledge practices to bear on health care, making its content visible in new and standardized ways. As an essential part of health care restructuring, health informatics links health care 'content' to formal structures of 'decision support,' transforming all aspects of the organizational design of health authorities. In new information-based methods of health care management and governance, decisions of every sort can be programmed to meet policy objectives,

This new information-based approach to managing health care addresses a long-standing and stubborn problem. Professional work in health care settings is notoriously difficult to manage, owing to the non-systematic work processes followed by its high-status participants. Medicine and medical practice are therefore the prime target for more objective management. The 'evidence' movement in medicine that Timmermans and Berg (2003) carefully appraise offers new possibilities for transcending complete reliance on individual professional judgement by bringing scientific research to bear systematically and accountably on physicians' diagnostic and treatment decisions. Uniform ways of knowing about patients, diseases, drugs, and other interventions and their results permit the identification of 'best practices' and can standardize how physicians make clinical decisions. Timmermans and Berg (2003) argue that evidence-based medicine (EBM) could improve both therapeutic effectiveness and the effective use of resources if evidence-based clinical guidelines were to be widely accepted and used. In spite of substantial difficulties in instilling clinical guidelines into professional practice, they remain optimistic about the benefits for health care that a wise use of standards offers, anticipating that evidence-based medicine will join forces with the quality improvement movement in hospital management.

Although nursing practice differs significantly from medical practice, science is an authoritative force to which nurses, as well as doctors, accede. The nursing profession generally accepts and endorses the premises of EBM and is integrating evidence-based practice into nursing (Ingersoll 2000; but also see Estabrooks 1998). Various notions of evidence carry a good deal of weight with nurses as they continually reassess how to act properly as professionals, employees, citizens, and workers in Canada's changing public health care system. Besides offering a guide for 'best practices' in both medicine and nursing, standardized, scientifically oriented, knowledge about health care makes an important contribution to new ways of routinizing, rationalizing, and comparing therapeutic regimens and broadening the reach of systems of managing professional practice.

The authority of evidence-based standards and their potential uses in a health care workplace must be considered within the long-standing interprofessional relations that organize nursing practice. In their study of physicians' evidence-based practices, Timmermans and Berg remain acutely sensitive to physicians' professional vulnerabilities and needs (e.g., for maintaining maximum discretion and flexibility within the use of clinical guidelines). When they mention nurses, it is often in that context, pointing out, for instance, how a more standardized medical practice is complemented by the redesign of medical secretaries', receptionists', and nurses' work. Although they see workplace changes that facilitate a standardized approach as sometimes enriching those new jobs, their attention is primarily focused on reorganizing work to protect physicians from the most routine and dull features of increasing the standardization of medical practice. Of course, the changes that would make evidence-based medicine successful both for gaining the acceptance of physicians and for improving the quality of health care are massively transformative of health care settings. Timmermans and Berg say that 'the world of medicine is "remade and molded" through standardization' (2003, 22). Nurses have been insisting for some time that they, too, must be involved in any remaking of health care, but the processes that are transforming it supersede professional knowledge and goals. We will be arguing here that quality improvement in health care increasingly relies on the expertise of information professionals, auditors, and managers who generate and use a different kind of expertise from that of health professionals. While they do not explicitly discuss the potential for the goals and aspirations of these different groups to conflict, Timmermans and Berg do recommend making space in the development of systems for the negotiation of just such issues. And they recognize that tensions exist between the benefits of standardization and the maintenance of sufficient flexibility to satisfy differently situated goals and values.

We want to take up something that is not addressed in the Timmermans and Berg analysis – the issue of standpoint. What is problematized in any study depends on the location and situated interests of the analyst. One of our interests in assessing health care's organizational strategies is to look at what works *for whom* in a system that is insured and administered publicly, that is, 'in the public interest.' Both expert knowledge and public mandates confer authority. In the settings that we research, conflicts over competing values emerge (or get squelched) as the capacity for control and coordination changes. It is no secret that nurses are located differently from physicians within the relations of the health care system. We cannot assume that what is true for doctors is also true for nurses. We want to sort out how standardized tools that are organizing the health care work processes are or might be experienced differently by differently located practitioners. It is possible that nurses might understand quite differently from either doctors or hospital managers what is a successful outcome or benefit of services provided. Our research approach, discussed later, maintains the capacity to recognize the importance of participants' different locations. Rather than submerging and overlooking such differences, we exploit participants' social location and standpoint. For instance, the application of evidence to medicine and the measurement of performance indicators in health care may indeed improve the care given. Whether or not they do, and when and under what circumstances, are empirical matters that deserve more analytic attention. Some serious issues emerge about whose definitions of improvement would be used in any such inquiry. We develop these ideas further as we show nurses caught up in standard organizational practices that sometimes contravene their own beliefs about good nursing.

Before we can discover what shifting organizational arrangements enter nurses' work and reconstitute elements of its routine character, we need to look more closely at some of the relevant features of public sector management. In this regard, we draw on a history of the implementation of public policy. We can learn, for instance, from research on the innovation of management in U.N. projects (Ilcan and Phillips 2003, 2005; Phillips and Ilcan 2003), research that considers critically the importance of information infrastructures for implementing and managing public policy. We were struck by the resemblance between these accounts of the development of technical expertise as an arm of U.N. policy implementation and the contemporary operation of Canadian health care reform and hospital restructuring.

Managerialism[5] in the Implementation of Public Policy

As we have suggested, in Canada the public responsibility for funding health care puts a strong focus on its proper administration. Public administrators must maintain an efficient, effective, and equitable system of delivering health care, while relying on the expertise of health professionals whose activities are not necessarily or fully under the control of the system. Historically, it has been the work of these same health professionals that constitutes (or not) its quality of care, effectiveness, and efficiency. One of the prevailing challenges of public health administration is how to access and put to effective use the expertise that a health care workforce currently monopolizes. Developing knowledge in appropriate forms makes possible a more systematic, rational and accountable operation of health care organizations. The enlistment of science to help make the world of health care knowable in standard ways plays an increasingly important part, not just for health care professionals, but also in health care administration and management.

Our analysis opens some of these administrative undertakings to systematic scrutiny. The studies that Suzan Ilcan and Lynne Phillips (2003) conducted in another policy arena in some ways mimic our interests in the Canadian health care field. For instance, Ilcan and Phillips show how technical expertise is key to the successful diffusion of public policy across vast geographic space and diverse political jurisdictions – as we do, regarding Canadian health care policy. They have studied the work of the United Nations and specifically the U.N.'s food and agricultural programs for the alleviation of global food scarcity. They discuss the new science-based approaches to food production and distribution that, from the middle of the twentieth century, were being planned and implemented worldwide. The goal was a rationalized, reorganized, and renewed system of food production to be put in place by local people whose work practices would also have to be reconceptualized, reorganized, and renewed. Through the Food and Agricultural Organization's technical expertise, food was 'informatized' (Ilcan and Phillips, 2005) by professional experts or technoscientists. Knowledge about a target nation's food, nutrition, crop production, food consumption, local food deficits, rules for the export and import of food stuffs, and so on was developed in standard forms. The ground (of participating countries, food production and use, the people and their nutritional needs) was 'mapped' in the terms given by the food information. As it became the basis for action authorized by the FAO and its associated agencies, knowing in standard ways conferred power. The range of food-related programs implemented would be those that this information described, justified, and authorized.

The comparisons to new processes of managing health care are striking. They advance our thinking about the connections between science, management, and both planned and unforeseen consequences. For our purposes, the key point here is that the model of governance innovated and used by the United Nations from its inception in 1945 requires and runs on specific, and specifically formatted, knowledge. About the knowledge generated, Ilcan and Phillips note the virtual invention of concepts and categories to render the subject area or population manageable: 'The generation of specific forms of knowledge and expertise remained integral to those processes ... that not only governed human capacities and acted upon them by technical means, but that mapped the different sites that could be governed in the name of progress and development' (1002: 442).

Hidden at the heart of this kind of governance is something that might mistakenly appear to be only a by-product of the work: the transformation of a setting that takes place *as information for its management is generated.* Ilcan and Phillips give a glimpse into the transformation of settings that occurs when expert accounts (expressing international interests within frameworks of scientific criteria) are substituted for local knowledge. They suggest that it happens as locals are trained, transferring into subject populations the 'standard' view, including how to properly measure and calculate food production, what crops are to be grown, their expected output, and how to accomplish these ends. Constructing how the setting is to be known reconstructs how it will be, and what it can become. The sites, the people, and the activities that were to be the subjects of the food policies not only *were transformed* in the process, they *had to be transformed* by the application of methods of measuring, coding, classifying, and standardizing them. Phillips and Ilcan point out that, regardless of this intensive mobilization of science, people remain 'stubbornly hungry' (2000: 448). It is not just the failure to prevent famine and suffering that worries these analysts but also the negative effects of the FAO activities that they see as colonizing local knowledge and practices. They conclude that 'such an approach not only homogenizes or ignores what is considered 'minor' or 'irrelevant' knowledge ... but promotes an indifference to difference by putting aside the possible significance of diverse practices' (Ilcan and Phillips 2005: 19). They reflect on the meaning of the losses, noting that whereas much diversity in the world has already been standardized out of existence, local practices, when retained, continue to be relevant, not just to local people, but even more widely as the value of diverse ecosystems is recognized. All this will have a recognizable ring to those, like us, who have been watching with a mixture of admiration and anxiety the changing environment of health care and its management in Canada.

Foreshadowed in this cautionary account of the methods that the United Nations was innovating in the post–Second World War period are the contemporary transformative technologies of the health care field. Do we similarly place too much hope in the potential of science and science-based management for improving health care? Does scientific medicine necessarily bring all the right solutions for the problems that interfere with people's health and well-being? What problems are being prioritized for attention? In health care, as in food production, only some problems will present themselves as 'the right kind of problem' to be solved (Ilcan and Phillips 2003: 446, citing Ferguson 1994: 70). But our aim is not simply to analogize the efforts and effects of the FAO to the health care setting. More importantly, and of more analytic usefulness, is how this study of the governance of global food production, distribution, and consumption directs our analytic attention to the (increasingly managerialist) technologies of management and governance in Canadian health care. Our inquiry focuses on similar issues that arise in health care when the subjects of its governance are constituted, reconstituted, and disciplined towards dominant goals.

Public administration in the industrialized world is itself being reformed by the so-called new public management whose practices carry into mature public service sectors a new philosophy, or at least new rhetoric, and a new set of management practices. Variously seen as guided by 'neo-liberalism' (Broadbent and Laughlin 2002), and as 'a movement' employing 'private sector styles of management' and a 'quasi-market' orientation (Dawson and Dargie 2002: 34–6), the new public management is expected to increase efficiency, reduce costs, and improve the quality of services, while reducing direct government involvement. The claims for the new public management are varied, and so are the pressures that motivate its adoption in different jurisdictions. The latter include economic pressures and high-level political and ideological commitment for change.[6] In Canada the pressure of 'global capital markets' on the federal government to eliminate the budget deficit in the mid-1990s is said to have encouraged some public sector reform (Borins 2002: 186). It triggered a good deal more at the provincial and regional levels. Reducing the federal budget deficit meant reduced transfer payments and constituted for the Canadian provinces a crisis of (health) funding for which restructuring, within strategies of the new public management, provided at least a partial solution.

Broadbent and Laughlin claim that the common feature of the new public management, at the level of public service provision, is its pervasive 'accounting logic.'[7] Expressed through a new managerialism in Canadian health care, an accounting logic generates the 'expression of outputs and outcomes linked to financial inputs' (2002: 105). But these British analysts of public administration are sceptical of the wholesale application of accounting logic in health administration. Quoting Gallhofer and Haslam (1991: 495) they say that 'expressed particularly through the technologies of accounting, [accounting logic] produces an aura of factual representation, promoting a general perception that it generates "neutral, objective, independent, and fair" information' (Broadbent and Laughlin 2002: 102). Carrying this concern forward into our own inquiry, we draw on a similarly critical analysis found in Geoffrey Bowker and Susan Leigh Star's 'fundamental rethinking of the nature of information systems' (1999: 321).

The Textual Representation of Health Care

In the restructured health care system, the provision of services is co-ordinated textually. The new methods, the accounting logic, and its managerial implementation require that the patients, nurses, and nursing be reformulated, calculated, and enumerated. The management of planning and resource allocation, programs of therapeutic interventions, and process and outcome monitoring take place on the basis of this textual representation; that is, they are worked up and worked on as virtual realities. And this has unforeseen consequences. As Ian Hacking says, 'enumerating requires categorization' and 'defining new classes of people for purposes of statistics has consequences for the ways in which we conceive of others and think of our own possibilities and potentials' (1990: 7). The new information makes what is known in one world knowable in language common to another, for instance, moving from the world of nursing to that of hospital management. New forms of classification and categorization make that sort of trans-literation appear natural, even when, as Ilcan and Phillips argue (2003 and elsewhere), they transform the world in the course of describing it.

Bowker's and Star's elaboration of this point about information construction makes an important contribution to our analytic framework. They challenge the naturalness of what they call 'built information landscapes' – organizational infrastructures composed of formal and commonsensical categories, standards, specifications, and classifications. Largely accepted and taken for granted in any organization, Bowker and Star insist that there are moral, ethical, and political implications 'when policy decisions are layered into inaccessible technological structures' (1999: 320). Information infrastructures accomplish the crucial, delicate, and always flawed task of constructing representations that straddle multiple worlds, connecting different contexts of practice. While categories and classifications may indeed 'make things work like magic' (1999: 9), Bowker and Star point out that 'each standard and each category valorizes some point of view and silences another' (1999: 5). We think it is important to apply that insight to nursing and ask, When nursing is represented in terms that make it objectively manageable, whose values are expressed and whose are silenced? Treating as natural the reformulation of nurses' knowledge into information for management uses may obfuscate something that, if made visible, might elicit a different practical response. Our research looks into circumstances in nursing where we argue that this is indeed the case. We must then confront the irremediable issue of multiplicity, of different views, and of the power advanced through the built-information landscape, as particular representations determine whose ideas and interests will be accepted and promoted.

Important decisions about health care rely heavily on the apparent objectivity and good sense of determining courses of action whose outcomes, benefits, success rates, cost comparisons across peer groups, and so on, have been numerically calculated. In this book we explore how, under new technologies of management and governance, nursing work processes are being brought into line objectively, rationally, and authoritatively with outcomes that have been predetermined elsewhere to be desirable and emblematic of success, including 'quality of care.' The activities and processes through which such coordination of knowledge, judgement, purposes, and action are organized have become our focus of inquiry. In the chapters that follow, we look more closely at such calculations and what they may mean in actual sites of nursing.

A Standpoint in the Everyday World

Our inquiry begins on the ground of health care – the actual stuff of interpersonal care being given by nurses in hospital settings. Beginning there, we focus on the social organization of nursing work within settings constituted through health care reform and the managerial practices that are transforming those settings. Health care is being restructured to solve certain problems. It is our claim that restructuring tackles problems as they are defined from a managerial viewpoint, and in doing so, other problems – that are experienced by nurses and patients, for instance – are overlooked. To develop this as an argument, we identify, illustrate empirically, and explicate how the health care system is being organized, not primarily for those it is expected to serve, but for what we show to be ruling purposes.[8]

The research approach we use is institutional ethnography (Smith 1987; 1999; Campbell and Gregor 2002). The idea in institutional ethnography is to explore 'how things work' from the standpoint of those who live the everyday experience, in this case, that of nurses having their work lives restructured. Using institutional ethnography, we identify the perspective embedded in the operation of the managerial technologies and the information resources that feed them. It is in these *practices* that nurses' work is coordinated with the calculation of costs and/or outcomes that constitutes the restructuring agenda and what we claim is a ruling standpoint. We make the assumption that ruling relations pervade nursing and health care as they do all other sites of governing and managing. Dorothy Smith (1999) introduces 'ruling relations' as a way of problematizing for empirical investigation what Bowker and Star, too, want not to be left unexamined – the organization and concerting of people's activities in processes that prior to such scrutiny would seem to be autonomous systems. Smith would say that the work-up of the everyday world into the virtual realities of classifications and categories is part of an historical trajectory of the development of the relations of ruling. In the present historical moment 'information, knowledge, reasoning, decision-making, "culture," scientific theorizing and the like become properties of organization' (Smith 1999: 78), seemingly displacing the actual people who exercise will and judgement. But people are there and they are active. Finding them, exploring what they do and how they are organized to do it is how an institutional ethnographer discovers ruling. Being ruled means that while actual people's own participation remains integral to all forms of organization, their actions are being regulated, and their individual will and judgement are systematically superseded. For instance, through the workings of classifications that Bowker and Star (1999) dissect, subject populations are socialized to become that which can be and is measured. And measurement is the crux of management. Michael Dector, while chair of the board of the Canadian Institute of Health Information (CIHI) said, 'If you can't measure it, you can't manage it' (CHSRF 2000: 6).

A statement such as Dector's can be accepted as unremarkably true only in a world that, Ian Hacking argues, has 'itself [become] numerical ... where numeracy is held to be as important as literacy' and where 'we have trained people to use numerals' to conceptualize and control everyday life (1990: 5). In a similar vein, Dorothy Smith points out the ubiquity of printed and electronic texts that mediate the 'intersection of everyday local settings and the abstracted, extra-local, ruling relations' (1999: 74). Our approach to organizational analysis addresses this intersection, and it does so by making analytical use of the texts that classify, enumerate, and administer nursing. In restructured health care settings this particular form of representation, and only this form, is positioned to be counted and acted on. Following Lucy Suchman (1993), who asked in another context how categories and their use are political, we explore empirically the textual organization of power in health care generally and in nursing particularly. In the chapters that follow, we examine some of the texts that hold expert knowledge of health care in categories, classifications, and so on, to see how, when, and by whom they are used. As we do, we keep asking and looking for answers to the question, Beside the taken-for-granted benefits of restructuring health care in this manner, what are the costs and to whom do they accrue? Beyond the potential for organizing and managing health care more systematically, we discover that hidden within the operation of these technologies there are new dangers to Canada's health care system, to nurses, and to patients, and these need to be better understood.

As we challenge ideas and practices that carry strong legitimacy within the health professions and the associated research community, our inquiry enters water that looks calm and troubles it. Health care reform, new approaches to the management of quality in health care, and hospital restructuring all appear to be addressing serious matters of public life, bringing needed innovations.[9] Similarly the imposition of accounting logic, whose everyday workings in health care we analyse, is not widely contentious,[10] remaining as Broadbent and Laughlin (2002: 106) say, 'substantially un-debated.' Clearly, we are not alone in criticizing the Canadian health care system, but our analysis opens up beliefs, practices, and states of affairs that appear, in the health care literature, as faits accomplis. The relevant discourses reflect the authority of scientifically validated, neutral, dominant practices and show the nursing profession to have adopted as its own the (ruling) perspective of health care restructuring. But there is another, largely subjugated, perspective.

In our inquiry, we take the standpoint of those who are subject to the restructuring of their workplaces and work processes. We want to 'tell the truth' from this standpoint (Smith 1999: 127). As institutional ethnographers, we analyse the text-mediated processes through which the big problems in health care are being defined, worked on, and apparently resolved. We find individual nurses participating in this work knowledgeably and conscientiously. One goal for our analysis has been to find out how nurses learn to be active practitioners of restructuring, and how they are active, as well, in altering nursing, often in ways that match neither their own nor their patients' interests. Learning about this brings us to the book's second major goal. We want to encourage Canadians to look again at so-called successful health care reform. We point out the danger inherent in treating as 'truth' the virtual reality that has been generated within and for the purposes of contemporary management practice. This is the knowledge relied on for constructing (or in this case, restructuring) health care. Our analysis offers many instances where objectified textual accounts of people's poor health and suffering and their care and treatment – the stuff of health care – may be adequately represented for the calculation of costs and benefits, but be deceptive about lives lived in the everyday world. Nurses work at the point of interchange between everyday life and its textual representation, and in coming to terms with nurses' involvement in the textualization of health care, we begin to see its implications. We understand these efforts to be ruling practice. As ruling practice, the textual representation supports the work of public policymakers, health planners, and accountants even when their interests are different from health care workers and patients.

In these textually mediated processes, a sophisticated form of power is exercised over nurses and their work. In studying nurses' restructured work, it becomes apparent that textually mediated ruling is a different form of power than that exercised by external authority over a passive or unwilling subject. Engaging in text-mediated work organizes nurses' consciousness, drawing them into the relevance of the text as subjects. They become the text's proponents, active in instituting the new order. Their standpoint is reorganized. But for nurses there is a contradiction. They remain in 'the everyday world' of patients and human interaction, where they continue to be confronted by the disquieting disjuncture between that actuality and the virtual realities constructed in managerial texts. It is that line of fault that our institutional ethnography explores and explicates.

The Structure of the Book

The book draws from several ethnographic studies undertaken separately by Janet Rankin[11] and Marie Campbell.[12] When we appear in the analysis as researchers, we follow the convention of being identified by our surnames. When we appear as participants or informants, we identify ourselves by our first names. Our argument begins in Chapter 1, where we describe health care reform both as it appears now, and from a longer perspective, in Canada. We argue that although the term reform has come into general usage in health care only since the early 1990s, the tensions that motivate use of contemporary restructuring technologies emerged long ago, even as the legislation instituting public health insurance was being passed in 1966. Then, as now, people worried about whether Canadians could afford public health care. Careful management of health care resources has been the aim of successive generations of nursing and hospital administrators. We focus on the efforts made in the 1960s, 1970s, and 1980s to improve the efficiency of hospitals through rationalizing the use of nursing labour. Patient classification – a technology used for representing, calculating, and rationalizing patient needs for nursing care – entered Canadian nursing during the 1970s and 1980s. It revolutionized nurse staffing and has provided the knowledge basis for the intensified management of nursing since then.

Chapter 2 explores the contemporary operation of one of the most widely used technologies of hospital management – a computerized program for keeping track of admissions, discharges, and transfers (ADT). We show that what might otherwise appear to be simply a technical tool for making the best and more efficient use of available hospital beds also organizes nurses to adapt their practice to its requirements. We identify ADT processes as integral to the new public management of health care – that operates on the basis of text-mediated knowledge linking patients and caregiving to management of the hospital's 'fixed investments.' New priorities emerge, including the emphasis on speeding up the movement of patients through the hospital, and as shown in the vignette we analyse, hurrying the patients out the hospital door. The virtual reality that ADT generates comes to dominate, even restructure, nurses' work, and this has a cost, not just for nurses themselves but for the care given to patients.

In Chapter 3 we introduce more managerial technologies that offer hospitals the capacity to make the therapeutic practices of caregiving more efficient. In clinical pathways, the steps that are taken to care for a patient with a particular condition are itemized and routinized to stabilize the patient's trajectory towards recovery and discharge. Another technology called alternate level of care (ALC) creates a routine process for sorting out 'appropriate' from 'inappropriate' patients who may occupy acute-care beds and absorb the level of nursing care routinely offered in acute-care wards. ALC creates the possibility to improve efficiency in the use of resources by delisting certain kinds of interventions for patients identified as 'inappropriate.' Our argument is that these objectifying technologies come to dominate nurses' own views and responses to patient care – and, of course, they are expected to do so. Nurses who activate the text-mediated processes that categorize patients learn to treat people as instances of the categories, absorbing as their own the perspective of restructuring with its valuing of 'efficiency.' It is our view that nurses' consciousness is restructured as they become agents of the restructuring technologies. We offer some observations of how this undermines patient care.

Chapter 4 inquires into the changing work of front-line nurse leaders under the new public management. The goals of a restructured hospital must be expressed in policies and strategies that add up to the more efficient use of nurses' time and of other resources. This means that contemporary front-line nurse leaders play a decidedly different role in nursing work than did head nurses – their predecessors in front-line supervision. The new leadership work is massively textual and organized in relation to technologies of management. Front-line nurse leaders are positioned to coordinate nurses' work with the new organizational goals, insisting that staff nurses recognize and accept their part in restructuring. The changing expectations of nurses in both leadership and direct care positions can occasion tension and conflict, and one such situation from our fieldwork offers an opportunity for us to reflect on some of the features of front-line nurse leaders' restructured work.

In Chapter 5 we look at how accountability in health care is a textual product distinct from what actually happens. The chapter begins with an ethnographic account of a hospitalized patient's care and the subsequent completion of a patient and family satisfaction survey. Janet Rankin accompanied a head-injured family member (her Aunt Hannah) throughout her hospitalization, acting as her family support and, in this case, also observing the nursing care given and reflecting on it in the posthospitalization survey. All these experiences provide the basis for our analysis of the intertextual complex that constitutes 'quality management' and its use of 'patient satisfaction,' 'patient-centred care,' and other strategies within a hospital. We show how constituting quality as a virtual object works within the new public management of hospitals, subordinating the standpoint of patients, families, and nurses. We argue that this form of accountability will not illuminate, let alone criticize gaps in care (such as Janet saw, in her aunt's case). We argue that accountability constituted within the new public management remains captured within the virtual knowledge that is being manufactured for ruling health care.

Our ethnographic data show nurses engaging in new textual practices that restructure health care workplaces and nursing itself – and even change how they talk about their work. In Chapter 6 we explore the use of language that mediates nurses' work relations, coordinating their consciousness with the managerial agenda. As exhibits, we analyse two texts of nursing scholarship, explicating how they exemplify this particular use of language and also how they promote a ruling perspective in nurse readers.

Having problematized how nurses *know* their work, we observed what our informants said and did as they engaged in ordinary sites of nursing practice. This book examines the social organization that ties nurses into courses of nursing action that become both sensible and necessary in reformed workplaces. It is our contention that when nurses' work is ordered in relation to the accounting logic of the health care system's new public management, nursing is restructured. In the book's Conclusion we consider what this means for nurses and for the Canadian public.

Not just nurses but everybody who believes in the value to Canadians of Canada's health care system should learn more about what happens when health care is managed more 'objectively,' when decisions about health care are or can be made from afar on the basis of specially constructed texts. Our analysis draws attention to the ruling standpoint expressed in such accounts. In spite of everyone's expectations of better management, certain new social costs are generated and people must absorb them. Nursing is a case in point. If nurses are to maintain their caring commitments, they must get a firm analytic grasp on how they are hooked into an accelerating wheel of so-called efficiency. They can understand the mystery of how they are drawn into activities inimical to their patients' care. Their location in the embodied world of patient care provides the essential experiential basis for nurses to know health care differently than through managerially authorized forms of knowledge. Canadians have always relied upon what nurses know to do for them when they are sick; now nurses' knowing makes another contribution. A standpoint in the everyday/everynight world informs a project of discovery and the making of alternative accounts that nurses and others can use. 'We want to *know* because we also want to act and in acting to rely on a knowledge beyond what is available to us directly' (Smith 1990a: 34). This book begins that project, by beginning with, but going beyond nurses' knowledge of their everyday / everynight experiences, and accounting for them analytically. In doing so, we recast what we all know about how health care works and suggest what we need to struggle over.

1 The Managerial Turn in Nursing

Health Care Reform and Nursing Efficiency

Medicare,[1] Canada's system of public health insurance, emerged slowly and indirectly out of citizens' post–Second World War demand for a more equitable distribution of resources. Money has always been at the centre of discussions about health care provision. Until Medicare was instituted, many Canadians couldn't afford health care. Government-subsidized hospital care was made available in 1957,[2] and by then some provinces were subsidizing private medical insurance for low-income people. In 1961, a fully subsidized system for insuring medical services was pioneered by the socially conscious government of Saskatchewan. It was taken up more or less completely in the policy platforms of successive federal governments, and in a climate of political turmoil, Medicare was finally legislated into existence as a national program in 1968. Provinces 'signed on' individually, under an agreement in which the federal government was to pay half of the associated costs. Under the Canadian funding system, and with no clear point indicating when intervention stops improving the health status of recipients, health care can absorb as much money as is made available. Management of the health care system, including keeping a lid on expenditures, is thus a necessary component of public responsibility. From the beginning, exercising this responsibility has been both complicated and highly contentious. What the system looks like today is the product not only of the original federal policy of required minimum standards,[3] but of Canada's federal-provincial-territorial decision-making.

This chapter focuses on these governments' early attempts to control one aspect of health care costs – the cost of nursing labour (Canada 1973). Support was provided for research that could predict and standardize how nurses spend their time in caring for hospitalized patients (MacDonnell 1968; Giovannetti et al. 1970; Giovannetti and McKague 1973; Equipe de Récherche Operationnelle en Santé 1978). Using such studies, management technologies were developed to substitute measurements and numerical projections for nurses' own professional decisions about patients' needs for nursing care (Campbell 1984; 1992; 1994). Measuring nurses' workload was the first step in allocating nurse staffing 'objectively.' Deploying nurses in relation to authoritative estimates of patients' needs was expected to help hospitals save money. It has, however, had much broader effects than that. The central thesis of this chapter is that shifting control over the definition of 'what patients need' is the basis for changing nurses' beliefs about their professional practice – including what constitutes adequate care. Of course, these changing beliefs have entered into the managerial project of cost control. How this has actually happened, and what it means that in recent years similarly 'objective' approaches to managing nursing have proliferated, are questions that capture our analytic attention throughout the rest of this book. We may agree that, while efficiency and good administration of funding are necessary, they are not the whole story. We attempt to balance that perspective by analysing how efficiency 'works' within nursing and what are its hidden costs.

Efficiency through Measuring and Accounting

Managing Canada's health care system is a complex undertaking, further complicated by intergovernmental relations – frequently characterized as 'squabbling.' The Canadian constitution gives provinces, and now territories, too, jurisdiction over health matters, with the federal government's influence over health care coming largely from its capacity to raise and deploy taxes. Provinces and territories establish and maintain their own delivery mechanisms for public not-for-profit health services, and they also string together other for-profit and privately operated programs and institutions, whenever they can argue that these additions meet the requirements of federal policy. Pressure to privatize health services, always the subtext of health care debates,[4] seems to be growing under initiatives to reduce the size of government and of government debt and deficits and to cut taxes and program spending in order to improve 'the climate for business investment' (Yalnizyan 2004: 2). Health care offers potentially lucrative business opportunities not just for investment in biomedicine and technology, but especially under new trade agreements, in the private management of the health service sector (see Fuller 1998, for a comprehensive and cautionary analysis). Even so, most Canadians continue to view public not-for-profit health care as a civic right, some going so far as to treat it as emblematic of our national identity.

Throughout the 1990s, health care came in for much public attention as provinces commissioned formal reviews of their systems in seeking ways to improve and sustain them.[5] Out of these reviews came recommendations that have fuelled more debate about the need for various reforms. Although Medicare remains popular with Canadians, the cost of delivering the services it designates is widely accepted as being too high, perhaps even unsustainably so.[6] The consensus for improving both the quality and the efficiency of the health care system tends towards managerial reform – towards implementation of strategies to use available resources more effectively. Common across the various provincial reviews, for instance, has been the idea that acute-care patients should be moved more quickly from institutions to their homes to recover, or if they are terminally ill, to be cared for there until they die. Motivating this idea were humanitarian concerns – returning sick people from institutional care to their community and family locale; furthermore as, well, this course of action was expected to help improve the utilization of expensive institutional resources.

Another impetus for health care reform came from the federal government's aggressive fiscal policy of deficit reduction that in the mid-1990s led to deep cuts in social spending. Federal transfer payments that supported the provincially run systems of health care were slashed. The original bargain to share costs equally between the federal and provincial governments had long since been abandoned, and with the fiscal restraint of the mid-1990s, the federal share sank in 1998–9 to a new low of about 10 per cent of health care dollars spent (Block 2004: 5). To maintain the 1990s level of services, the remaining 87 per cent of health care costs had to be picked up by the provinces and territories, in their capacity as administrators of the actual health care systems. Canada's provinces and territories responded to this demand in various ways, depending to some extent on their own political ideologies. Across the country a mixture of hospital mergers and closures, bed closures, staffing and program reductions, and privatization schemes were instituted (Dickenson 1996; Burke and Greenglass 2000). The resulting squeeze on services meant that health care became difficult to gain access to reliably in some places, and staff morale (Woodward et al. 1999) and patient care deteriorated (Armstrong et al. 2000). In Toronto, under a provincial government determined to cut social spending, health care went from bad to worse, so much so that the public media began reporting cases of emergency departments filled to overflowing and ambulances being turned away. Everywhere, according to media reports, waiting lists for surgery were growing.[7] Presumably in response to public criticism, both the federal Liberal government and a standing committee of the Canadian Senate sponsored extensive inquiries (Romanow 2002; Kirby 2002)

At the same time as the federal government was implementing its policy of deficit reduction, it was reorganizing how state-sponsored research, including medical research, would be funded. New expectations for medical research (now called health research) were being proposed. For instance, in Canada, as elsewhere, research findings were to inform health care practice expeditiously, thus avoiding the waste of precious resources on ineffective treatments.[8] How to accomplish this transfer of findings (later called knowledge translation) was itself a new topic for health research. Generous grants for knowledge transfer and translation were made available through the new Canadian Health Service Research Foundation (CHSRF)[9] and the Canadian Institutes of Health Research (CIHR)[10] for improving the efficiency and effectiveness of Canadian health care by determining how to get that knowledge used and establishing methods for measuring results. Health research expanded to include funding for research that was specifically administrative and relevant to decision-makers' needs. Through the Canadian Institute for Health Information (CIHI), this new direction for research supported and indeed, even helped constitute what is being called the era of accountability in health care.[11] This approach developed and tested indicators to be used in measuring the performance of hospitals and their staffs or the satisfaction of patients and for choosing the appropriate patient from a waiting list, among many other newly minted managerial functions. Rendering more and more aspects of health care available to managerial scrutiny and comparison was becoming the basis for redesigning and improving the health care system's efficiency.

Debate about how to solve the multifaceted 'crisis in health care' continued to gather momentum at the turn of the millennium. On the political scene, health care dominated federal-provincial-territorial discussions. It became a bellwether in the ongoing disputes over legal jurisdiction and authority that a pending change in federal government leadership, finally realized in 2003, brought to a head. Regardless of variously argued positions on the benefits of private versus public services and the acceptability of introducing for-profit health care, everybody seemed to agree on one thing – that health services could and should be reformed. Within hospitals, the development of new and improved means of managing everything from patient flow to clinical treatment decisions was creating something of a revolution in the practice of health care. This is often talked and written about as 'restructuring.' While the literature addresses restructuring as an organizational topic, it has implications for and effects everybody involved – hospital administrators and information professionals certainly, but also physicians, nurses, and technicians, as well as cleaning, clerical, and kitchen staff, and – not least – patients and their families.

All this discussion about reform and restructuring would suggest that interest in improving the efficiency of Canadian health services was a new concern; not so. Elimination of waste has always been central to good management, in health care as elsewhere. Efficient utilization of resources was the reason that health policymakers as early as in the 1960s looked at the utility of measuring *needs* for health services to replace public *demands*. These efforts intensified over the years and still plague planners. Eminent health economist Robert Evans (1984) in discussing the complexities of health care suggests that it is nearly impossible to correlate people's health status with the level of health care intervention – which is how an economist would determine 'efficient' use of resources. Nor does Evans believe that for-profit organization and its built-in pressure for profit maximization would ensure for health care provision the same minimization of costs as it does in capitalist production, given the many differences between providing health care and the production and sale of other commodities. Yet for some time analogies of that sort of bottom-line thinking about public sector management have featured in the health care management literature (e.g., Robbins 1984). Currently, methodologies imported from the private sector, the new public management, are changing the culture of the public sector (McLaughlin, Osborne, and Ferlie 2002; Thomas 1996). Consider McCoy's account of the documentary practices that she sees as central to the new public management. She says the purposes of the new public management's documentary practices are to '*discover* and *represent* in calculable and comparable terms relevant administrative *objects* such as measurable inputs and outputs, unit costs, transaction volumes, rates of error or wastage, length of time for service delivery, customer satisfaction, efficiency ... that as a class of documentary practices are called "performance indicators"' (1999: 9–10, emphasis added). Our analysis in this chapter and this whole book reflects on what it means for health professionals to be part of this process of objectification.

The new public management of the1990s elaborates, and applies to many more aspects of health care provision, the kind of documentary management processes that we saw emerging much earlier. The 1970 *Report of the Review of the Costs of Health Services* (vol. 1, 43–5) had recommended attacking waste on several fronts, including what was seen as nurses' overgenerous use of their time spent in caring for patients. Nursing labour was a significant part of a hospital's budget, and unionization of increasing numbers of nurses in the 1970s was adding to labour costs. Already under way by then were the research projects that would more precisely describe and time nursing tasks to create a technology called patient classification. Research such as carried out by the Saskatchewan Hospital Systems Study Group (Sjoberg and Bicknell 1968) studied nursing in situ and quantified, abstracted, standardized, and reconceptualized the new object: 'patients' needs for nursing care.'

Patients' needs for nursing care were being classified into definite and recognizable levels. Once patients' needs for nursing care could be conceptualized in commensurable terms, hospitals (and their expenditures on nursing labour) would be less reliant on individual nurses' judgements about the amount of care that should be provided. Measurements of this sort made possible more objective allocation of nursing staff. This technology was adopted extraordinarily quickly,[12] offering as it did one avenue for hospitals to more effectively manage the funding crisis that the 1977 Established Programs Financing Act[13] had created.

Nurse staffing had been imprecise prior to the advent of the staffing methodologies that patient classification made possible.[14] Decisions about how many nurses a hospital would hire as regular employees and how many would be assigned to work, shift by shift, depended upon accumulated historical experience. Patient censuses were the only hard data available on which to modify the historical staffing complement for a ward. This census information, however, told how many beds were filled but revealed nothing about patient acuity (how ill a patient is). That meant that census information could not be used to discriminate effectively among differing levels of staffing needed in wards with the same number of patients. The expected 'hills and valleys' in patients' needs for care that occurred daily were identified as wasteful of nurses' paid time, even though the number of nurses assigned to a hospital ward reflected what nurses had always considered a workable ratio between patients and nurses. Staffing decisions were the responsibility of the nursing administration, and there was little flexibility, even though supervisors kept a close watch over patients' progress in order to offer a 'float nurse' as an extra pair of hands when necessary. On such a request from a head nurse to her nursing supervisor, staffing might be temporarily increased. That meant that head nurses' judgements about the intensity of any day's work were the best source of expertise available.

Head nurses would, of course, have individual and varying ideas about the amount of care necessary, how fast nurses could or should be asked to work, and so on, that would temper their decisions about asking for 'extra staff.' They would also have varying capacities to make nurses work quickly, and hospital administrators had no objective information about which head nurses were more successful in this regard. Such arrangements gave hospital administrations very little control over the nursing labour force and its productivity. Unlike forms of work where tasks are precisely specified, hospital administrators had no influence over nurses' ideas about 'good care,' and how to give it, or over their commitment to giving care efficiently. Even when policymakers could identify the problems that this incapacity caused, hospital administrators lacked the technical capacity to take charge. All this began to change in the 1970s. We turn now to a more detailed discussion of how these growing concerns played out in the development and use of a technology that specified nurse staffing allocation more precisely. And we begin to consider how, over time, this and other management technologies have substantially altered the practice of nursing.

Classifying Patients' 'Needs': A Technology of Resource Allocation.

We rely here on a study conducted in one Canadian hospital in the early 1980s that analysed how patient classification reformulated what nurses did with their time in the name of good nursing care.[15] As in efforts to apply management technologies elsewhere, nursing, too, had to be worked up conceptually to make it objectively manageable. For the reasons suggested above, nursing and particularly nurse staffing were logical targets for standardization and the objective management it facilitated.[16] The managerial achievement of classifying patients was to stabilize the meaning of patients' needs for nursing care. The autonomy nurses had exercised previous to this time over what patients needed in nursing care became a problem that was to be solved by more effective hospital management.

In hindsight, it is easy to see the revolutionary significance of patient classification that was being introduced into nursing. Classifications, according to Bowker and Star, are 'tools that are both material and symbolic' (1999: 286), ones that play a significant part in how large-scale bureaucracies work. Classifications represent conceptually the experience gained in one time and one place so that it can be linked with experience in another time and another place, and that is especially useful in management systems that attempt to regularize the movement of information between contexts. Here it is applied to nurses. Through information generated in the classification system, nurses' work was being regularized: standard 'classes' of patients require standard efforts. Features of patients' clinical presentation (confusion, pain, incontinence, reduced mobility, treatments, and so on) that led nurses to make certain choices about their care were identified, classified and standardized (see Figure 1.1). About this work, Bowker and Star (1999: 291) remind us that 'in order to be meaningful, [different] contexts of information must be re-linked through some sort of judgement of equivalence or comparability.' With patient classification, individual nurses' judgements about care for individual patients (in multiple hospital wards across Canada) were being relinked to standard times for caring for similar patients in research sites. In each of these new hospital wards, patients' needs for care were made equivalent, one patient to the next, one ward to the next.

The classification of patients generated something entirely new for nurses – an authoritative reading of the *time required for their work* that was made within a management process. Providing the knowledge basis[17] for new objective staffing methodologies, patient classification came to replace nurses' professional knowledge and judgement and in the process devalue nurses' knowledge as being 'subjective.' Patient classification established as authoritative its account of 'patients' needs for care' through being generated 'scientifically' and sponsored by a hospital's administrative hierarchy. This points to a feature of classifi-

Figure 1.1: Patient Classification

UNIT: ______________ TEAM: ______________ TODAYS DATE: ______________

For Full Description of Care - Please See Guidelines

Rater: ______________

Direct Nursing Care in 24 Hrs.

Time Values:
Factor 1 - 30 min.
Factor 2 - 30-60 min.
Factor 3 - 60-120 min.
Factor E3 - over 120 min.

		PERSONAL CARE				NUTRITION			ACTIVITY			TEACHING & EMOTIONAL SUPPORT			TREATMENT OBSERVATION							
		SELF CARE	ASSISTANCE	COMPLETE CARE	OVER 120 MIN. REQUIRED/24 Hrs.	MINIMUM ASSISTANCE	PARTIAL ASSISTANCE	NEEDS TO BE FED	MINIMUM SUPPORT	REQUIRES ASSISTANCE	FULLY DEPENDENT	0-30 Min./24 Hrs.	30-60 Min./24 Hrs.	60-120 Min./24 Hrs.	0-30 Min./24 Hrs.	30-60 Min./24 Hrs.	60-120 Min./24 Hrs.	OVER 120 Min./24 Hrs.	TOTAL			
																			1	2	3	PAT.CLASS
Rm. No.	Patients Name	1	2	3	E3	1	2	3	1	2	3	1	2	3	1	2	3	E3				

TOTALS	Team Sub Total	1	2	3	4	5	Team Census
	Combined Totals	A	B	C	D	E	Unit Census

cation that Bowker and Star want information designers and users to recognize: that technical decisions made in the design of classifications systematically reflect 'organizational and political positions' (1999: 322–3). Across contending and politically sensitive views, patient classification becomes information that renders stability of meaning to the amount of time needed to nurse standard classes of patients. It is in that technical sense that the information is 'objective.'

To be instituted, patient classification requires nurses' active cooperation. Indeed, it was nurses who activated the texts that 'classified' their patients. Strategies to ensure nurses' cooperation were carefully planned in the hospital that was studied and in others where the technology was being introduced. A carrot-and-stick approach was used to increase nurses' receptivity. The 'carrot' was the claim made for measuring workload through classifying patients – that when the acuity of their patients' conditions was properly represented by classifications, nurses would find staffing levels adjusted and, when necessary, increased. This made sense to nurses for a number of reasons. Many were experiencing cuts to their staffing, and nurses would be all too frequently 'working short' – with fewer than designated staff. Also, when there was no comparative information, nurses were always wondering if their ward was getting its proper share of the available nursing workforce. Patient classifications seemed to offer equity in this regard.

Implementation strategies were also used to get 'buy-in' from the nurses whose cooperation was needed. Head nurses, especially those who had a good reputation among their peers and were respected by staff nurses, were recruited to work up and test the local application of the classification system (also see Willis 2004). Nurses in Campbell's (1984) study were encouraged to revise the wording of the classification form and to add new categories, and so on, so that they could be satisfied that it accurately reflected the important aspects of their care for patients. It remains unclear whether this attention to adapting the tools to incorporate nurses' language was a misrepresentation of how classification would work – against them – or whether it was just naivety among nurses at lower levels in the nursing hierarchy. At any rate, it appears to be absolutely the case that management's purpose in introducing patient classification was to reduce spending on nursing labour, already identified by policymakers as being too generous.

The 'stick' that supported implementation was 'responsibility budgeting,' newly introduced to nursing units in the 1970s. Under responsibility budgeting (which preceded nursing units being treated as 'cost centres'), hospitals made head nurses responsible for their staffing budgets. This had the effect of making head nurses into managers with an organizational interest in getting more work out of their staff. Patient classification and its related staffing methodologies were a boon to head nurses whose own effectiveness in their jobs now depended upon learning to manage their unit budgets effectively. Classification was a powerful managerial tool because it made possible for the first time the objective calculation and enforcement of productivity expectations, that is, how much work a nurse is expected to get through in a day. If a nurse found it difficult to cope with her assigned work, now there was a standard to which she could be compared. Nurses began to find themselves being criticized as slow workers. Head nurses, whose effectiveness was judged by how well they managed tight budgets couldn't afford to hire or retain nurses who were or were likely to be slow. Head nurses had to see to it that nurses speeded up. Nurses learned that to satisfy the new demands of their jobs, as expressed by their head nurses, they had to work differently.

Of course, for nurses being pulled into the classification technology in the early 1980s, the classification system itself was not seen as a very important issue, given what they were up against at work when nurse staffing was inadequate. Nurses were told, and they continued to believe, that classifying patients would help identify the correct staffing numbers and that this would result in sufficient nurses appearing on a shift to get the work done. Nurses engaged in certain forms of negotiation around classifications – both authorized and unauthorized. Occasionally, if all the nurses on a unit were in agreement that the workload exceeded their ability to cope, they would lobby for an adjustment in the system. For instance, on the burn unit where Janet Rankin was working in 1980, the nurses lobbied to increase the standardized units of time allocated to the category 'wound dressing,' arguing that burn dressings were more complex and time-consuming than other surgical dressings. Certain kinds of 'gaming'[18] of the classification numbers also occurred. For instance, according to Rankin, before auditing of nurses' classification was routinely done, a nurse might classify a patient who was slightly vague as 'confused' or someone who needed assistance to bathe as 'total care.' Ordinarily, however, nurses treated filling out the classification form as merely another bureaucratic task.

As the patient classification form was completed, it put in motion a process whose usual outcome was to justify the status quo, not make an increase to existing staffing levels. Nurses may have known that the number of staff made available was a reflection of what they had reported in their patient classification forms. But the structure of decision-making remained unclear to them and the staffing decision itself, mysterious. Because the system was officially sanctioned, and built on what they themselves had reported, nurses were implicated in a manner that bound them to its staffing outcome. It mattered to their work. Nurses assigned to a shift had to accomplish the work represented in the prospective calculations of their patient assignment, regardless of how much more work they might find actually needed doing to adequately care for these patients. They were stuck with 'making do.'

What becomes apparent after several decades is that nurses have readjusted their traditional beliefs about patients' needs, bringing them more into line with the less generous realities of hospital funding. Patient classification systems helped to accomplish that and then faded into the infrastructure, all but forgotten by the current generation of nurses who are unlikely to recognize or understand them. Here we want to consider how that could happen: how nurses' knowledge about their patients could be transformed into objectified information, and then into organizational decisions that are part of management technologies, and then, how those practices could be routinely forgotten or 'naturalized.' 'Naturalization' means 'stripping away the contingencies of an object's creation and its situated nature. A naturalized object has lost its anthropological strangeness. It is in that narrow sense de-situated – members have forgotten the local nature of the object's meaning or the actions that go into maintaining and recreating its meaning' (Bowker and Star 1999: 299).

Nursing in the Everyday World of the 1981 Hospital

The following vignette, from ethnographic data collected in 1981, describes a nurse negotiating the contingencies of the work she faced during one very routine morning on a hospital ward. We offer this to highlight the actualities of a nurse's work prior to the implementation of contemporary efficiency measures.

A Registered Nurse is assigned six patients, one of whom is going to the operating room around 8:30 a.m. The other patients include three of the sickest on the unit, assigned to her because they require RN care; her co-worker on this end of a nursing unit is a Registered Nursing Assistant. The RN, therefore, is responsible for the physical care of three patients who need bed-baths and close supervision of intravenous therapy and surgical wounds being drained with suction. As well, she has two patients who need assistance with their personal care. The RN must change dressings and check and change IV infusions for the RNA's patients, too. Her morning's work is carried out in the following manner. She gets the shift-change report and prepares her OR-bound patient; she takes the temperatures of all her patients, prepares those who will be eating breakfast, and does other early morning nursing procedures. This brings the time to 8:30, when the breakfast cart arrives.

Although it is not an 'RN function,' the Registered Nurse helps the RNA hand out breakfast trays to all the patients. The RN explained why it is impor-

tant to do this, saying 'on our unit, we work very cooperatively. It's not an RNA function to hand out trays either, and if I'm expecting her to come and help me make a bed, then I have to share this unprofessional job with her.' This takes until 8:45 when, as scheduled, the RN goes off the unit for her coffee break, arriving back to take up her morning care shortly after 9:00 a.m.

The RN now has two-and-a-half hours before her scheduled lunch break to finish her morning care. But her co-worker is away from the floor for the first 15 minutes as is the RN from the other end of the unit. So, she answers callbells from all the patients at her end of the unit and is available for emergencies in the other end. On the return of her co-worker from coffee, she finishes carrying out a request from one the RNA's patients, and then finds each of the returning nurses to communicate to them messages that she has received during their absence. In the meantime, she has handed basins to her own two patients who are well enough to wash themselves with assistance.

It is now 9:30. The RN checks and changes several IVs and checks the abdominal (or other) drainage and suction equipment that these patients have in place. She finds one patient in pain and in need of medication at a time when the unit's medication nurse is not available. The RN prepares, gives, and records an injection for relief of pain. She returns to her 'bathing with assistance' patients, rewarms their bath water, and washes their backs. She then helps each of them to sit at the edge of the bed, do deep breathing and coughing, and helps them stand and walk about the room and then to sit in chairs. It is now 10 o'clock. While the RN is making beds, she is interrupted by a request from her RNA co-worker who needs advice about a surgical drain. A surgeon has been in to inspect her patient's wound and has left the dressing open. The RN sees that the wound needs a change of dressing immediately, so she does it. The RNA helps by finishing the RN's bed-making and then assisting those patients back to their beds.

At 10:30, the RN begins bathing one of her sickest patients. She needs help to turn him and to change his bedding, so she goes to find the RNA. On her way, she looks in on her other sickest patients, changing an IV in the same trip. Upon her return, she finds the physician visiting; she has to remove her bath materials to help him examine the patient before being able to get back to her own tasks. At 11 o'clock, having finished working with the first bed-bathed patient, the RN surveys her remaining work. There is not enough time to do two bed-baths; the beds of both these patients look untidy, but one patient is resting quietly while the other is restless and complaining. She checks these two patients' surgical dressings, which were supposed to have been changed this morning. Her priorities require that the personal care (bathing and bed-making) be completed, leaving dressings until after lunch. Although the doc-

tor had ordered the dressings changed three times a day, the RN's prioritizing reduces this number of changes to two. She decides to sponge the restless patient, change his dressing, and make his bed. She finishes just in time to leave on schedule for the first lunch break, which is at 11:30.

Classifying Patients to Standardize the Work

How would the patient classification technology make sense of this nurse's experience of her patients and their requirements for care? The way that patient classification works is by representing each patient on a nursing ward as 'having' a standard need for a nurse's care. The research behind the documentation becomes part of the technology to *predict* the nursing care times needed for actual hospitalized patients. In becoming a textual representation, the actualities of patients and their care are expressed abstractly. In the hospital where Campbell conducted these ethnographic observations, the work-up of patients into classifications, and then into workload units, and finally into discrete staffing allocations was a procedure that began with nurses' own working knowledge of patients and continued in a text-mediated, partially automated, management-operated process. The work-up of the patients into classifications occurred the day before the predicted shift. Writing on a nursing worksheet (Figure 1.2) a nurse from the earlier shift accomplishes the first level of abstraction. She records her nursing judgement about each patient into the worksheet's categories.

Then to classify them, each patient's worksheet is consulted. The worksheet shown here in Figure 1.2 is adapted from a textual tool commonly used by nurses to hold and pass on nursing information to other nurses. Here its adaptation provides information in categories matching those of the patient classification form. Thus, under Personal Care (see Figure 1.1) a nurse might record 'self,' 'assist,' or 'total,' depending upon her knowledge of the actual care the patient has received that day. That becomes available to the classifying nurse whose work leads further towards a determination of how much care is needed for a patient and how much it will cost in terms of units of nursing time. Looking at Figure 1.1 (Patient Classification), we see the related times in the section on Personal Care, for instance. Patients ticked as being 'self-care' require between one and thirty minutes of personal care from the nurse in a shift.

In this manner, nurses' work becomes known about authoritatively through the patient classification system – as a textual abstraction, not the details of what each nurse will actually need to do. Whereas nurses

Figure 1.2: Nurses' Worksheet (Text from Sides One and Two)

NURSES' WORKSHEET (TO BE COMPLETED IN PENCIL)									
DIAGNOSIS: SURGERY: DOCTOR: CONSULTANT:									
DIAGNOSTIC TESTS					MEDICAL ALLERGY				
ORDER DATE	TEST	DATE DONE	ORDER DATE	REORDER	MEDICATION	DOSE	ROUTE	TIME	D/C

DATE	DAILY CLASSIFICATION						DIAGNOSIS:
							DOCTOR:
VITAL SIGNS					DATE:		
T.P.R.:	APEX:				I.V. THERAPY		
B/P							
INTAKE:	OUTPUT:						
OTHER:							
PERSONAL CARE: SELF☐ ASSIST☐ TOTAL☐							
					TREATMENT/THERAPY		
ACTIVITY: SELF☐ ASSIST☐ TOTAL☐							
NUTRITION: SELF☐ ASSIST☐ TOTAL☐							
DIET:							
FOOD ALLERGY:							
ELIMINATION SELF☐ ASSIST☐ TOTAL☐					TEACHING NEEDS:		
OTHER:							
					DISCHARGE PLANS/LONG TERM GOAL		

would previously arrive at work and engage with various elements of the situation, including the actual patients, to determine what needs doing, now a workload index (calculated from classifications)[19] has already established quasi-boundaries around the required work. Those boundaries around the work time are indirectly communicated to the nurse through her patient assignment, insofar as the time available for nursing work is specified (in the staffing decision). The staffing methodology determines the number of nurses to be assigned to a ward by processing the workload index with information from the nursing labour budget (as taken up in the next section).

The above vignette begins to suggest how calculating the time required to take care of each patient's needs, even if everything that needs doing is expressed accurately in the classification and is timed correctly, still doesn't account for nurses' work. Nursing work on a hospital ward is a different matter from what can be expressed by adding up each patient's needs individually, although these are the elements of nurses' work that are most easily measured.[20] If we return to the 1981 nursing morning, we can see something about individual patients' needs and how they relate to the total work. For instance, the RN's six patients are indeed her prime responsibility, but her RNA team-mate's six patients are also hers to oversee. The RN is also a member of the nursing team for the whole ward, with responsibilities related to the whole. Among the many things that the patient classification's textual representation of 'the required care' keeps out of sight is the sharing of the work and its finely choreographed negotiation. The contingencies of the work that remain unaccounted for include the unpredictable ringing of call-bells, the cooling and rewarming of bath water, the medication nurse being unavailable when needed, the surgeon arriving to assess a wound at an awkward moment. Notice, too, even in 1981, how adept the RN is at dropping out pieces of what would have been 'necessary' work – in this case, a treatment ordered by a physician. In this moment of nursing prioritizing we can glimpse both the beginning of, and the future potential for, a major reordering of the patient care in today's hospitals. In later chapters we identify some of the systematic changes that have occurred. Even in this 1981 description, however, the whole of a nurse's morning work seems entirely different from how its parts might have been represented.

Campbell discovered other problems in the representation of patients' needs through patient classification, too. An archeology of this particular technology, patient classification, shows how it works as a management strategy. Displacing nurses' knowledge of what patients need offers a powerful means of managing the cost of nursing labour. Economical staffing decisions depend both upon the way that 'needs' are reconstructed through patient classification and upon how those data are manipulated with budget information.

Objectifying Processes Reformulate 'What Nurses Know'

The patient classification form refers backward to the research that cor-related 'needs for care' with nursing time and forward to staffing calcu-lations undertaken in the hospital that Campbell studied. Both the background research and the daily textual work-up of patients into patient classifications reshape what nurses know about their patients and their work. Examination of the patient classification text itself makes it possible to trace its action in these two directions. Its origin in research is important to how it is applied and what it accomplishes in a workplace, even though, as already argued, even the best patient clas-sification form fails to capture and express exactly what patients need. 'No classification system can reflect either the social or the natural world fully accurately,' as Bowker and Star reiterate (1999: 323). But such precision is not necessary to make the technology work effectively. Campbell's analysis (1994) shows that when actual patients are described using averaged, standard times to represent the work they need, both patients and nurses are standardized. To put this another way, use of the technology assumes that patients have standard needs, and staffing levels are determined thereby. That is the dominating fea-ture. The patient classification calculations establish standard amounts of time needed for nursing; staffing decisions made in response to those calculations *require nurses* to act as if their patients' needs were indeed standard. Staff deployment that exactly matches the allocated hours of paid nursing work to the patient classification calculations would rou-tinely underestimate the work for reasons intrinsic to classification – its averaging and standardization of timed tasks. But a further economy is being accomplished much more insidiously. To understand it, we must trace how the patient classification information entered decisions for allocating staff. It entered as an abstraction, which is the only way that mathematical calculations can be conducted. In the hospital under study, a management-defined (and flexible) staffing formula[21] trans-ferred into the nurse staffing allowance any reductions in the nursing labour budget that the hospital decided upon. The flexibility was accomplished through having one term in the staffing formula 'y,' rep-resent any work nurses needed to do, or time they needed to spend, *outside* what the classification measured. Called 'indirect care,' its value was determined arbitrarily at the management level.[22] Across Canada, wherever patient classification was being introduced as a staffing methodology, consultation among nurse leaders occurred about what percentage of their time should be allotted for the many and sundry activities not accounted for in direct measurements of patient care – the foundation of the patient classification formulas. Regardless of what percentage of nursing time was identified, the 'indirect care' or the 'Y' term of the formula became an arbitrary managerial application. When the hospital wanted to reduce the amount of budget spent on nursing labour, the value of 'Y' in the formula would be reduced, thus reducing the paid time made available for all nursing care. Unbeknownst to nurses, who were reassured to know that the staffing calculation took into account the unpredictable part of their work, a hospital's management could cut its funding for nursing and feed that cut directly into nurse staffing, spreading it 'equitably' across the hospital.

The staffing formula brings the relevant information together to manage nurses. Processing a hospital's budget with patient classification information made new surveillance of nurses' productivity possible. As early as 1981, in the hospital studied by Campbell, a heightened productivity expectation increased the pressure on nurses to work harder, increase their pace of work, and be economical with their use of time. Hospitals could and did set presumptive productivity expectations for nurses that the staffing decisions implemented. As professionals, nurses take as their own responsibility the additional cost of completing their assigned patients' care when less time is allocated in which to do it. In this manner, nurses' work is treated as indefinitely expandable.

When less time is made available for the total care of their patients, not only do nurses speed up, but they work on unpaid time, according to the nurses Campbell interviewed. Another effect of this organized pressure on nurses' time is that nurses curtail the range of services and attention they give to patients. They individually reassess what to do for them. They have to priorize, as we saw in the above vignette. This is a professionally sanctioned method of nursing decision-making. As part of their trained competencies, nurses manage their own use of time by discriminating between more or less crucial nursing actions. In situations where they increasingly are faced with insufficient time to do everything that they think is necessary, nurses begin to revise downward what they consider to be necessary. Such prioritizing judgements are themselves work that requires nursing knowledge, skill, and attention to detail, as illustrated in the ethnographic observations of a morning's routine care that were collected in 1981.

Knowing the Work from the Ground Up vs Knowing 'Objectively'

The vignette above suggests that even if patient classification were to accurately describe classes of patients and their needs, it would not express the demands that meet nurses when they go to work. The classification projects an estimate of work, a textual reality, that is generated daily and in advance about a patient population that is extremely changeable. All sorts of complications occur on the ground to undermine the accuracy of that estimate. For one thing, the classification measures workload associated with a definite population of patients, but that list is rapidly outdated as hospitals move patients in, through their facilities, and out again as quickly as possible. Patients' conditions change all the time. Besides those located 'in' the patients, there are other variations related to the nursing setting. Time studies of nursing have been most successful in reflecting those aspects of the work nurses do directly with patients. But nurses' work is by no means limited to the bedside. They organize and coordinate an environment that houses patients and has many aspects that are similar to running a hotel. Nurses work in concert with a variety of auxiliary service providers, as we have glimpsed in the vignette. They provide a supportive environment for the practice of medicine, articulating their caring work to physicians' orders and practical needs. Another invisible but essential responsibility that nurses carry is the management of the patient's whole therapeutic regimen, including organizing his or her movements to other hospital departments for special treatments and the like. Nurses are involved with the public, communicating with families and other visitors, some of whom need special attention, instructions, and interpretation. These and many other background tasks, apparently peripheral but actually necessary to the adequacy and flow of care take nurses' time, and it is time over which nurses do not exercise effective control. These indeterminate features of the work are given quantitative expression in the patient classification, thereby 'hardening' the figures it generates. But the apparent precision in matching needs (that relate to defined work) to staffing (expressed as paid time) that the system offers is reduced by all these possible variations not captured in the textual version. This allows staffing decisions to appear adequate when they are not. Then it is over to the nurses on duty to 'make do.' Making decisions about cutting out some of the nursing care that their patients actually need relies on nursing judgement. As a direct consequence of patient classification, nurses began during the 1970s and 1980s to have to make such important decisions as a matter of everyday routine and usually on the run.

Under this early management technology nurses retained discretion – a feature of their professional work organization in which the practitioner chooses how to apply his or her knowledge and skills – in relation to each patient. Although, under patient classification, the patient's nursing regimen is codified in texts, *how* that work gets done – the specificity of each generally designated task, the sequence in which tasks are undertaken, the attention to detail required (for instance, in carrying out asepsis) – is not defined. (That changes during the next decades, as we shall see in later chapters.) Decisions about what care can be hurried over, skimped on, or deleted completely are left to nurses.

The work of nurses has, as well, the character of women's work, in which women 'pick up the pieces' of whatever needs to be done to advance a project.[23] Hospital units are particularly reliant on nurses seeing what needs doing and doing it, and seeing what is going wrong and correcting it, even if it is not in their job description (see Campbell 2000). All of these features of nurses' actual work make something of a mockery of the attention previously given to measuring and matching needs and work so precisely. Yet the patient classification calculation stands as an expression of an objectively correct relationship between the nursing care to be provided and the quantity of work that is considered necessary and to be paid for. It is our view that the appearance of objectivity about this previously professional judgement produces the key achievement of patient classification as management technology. In the 1980s, in hospitals all over Canada, this objective calculation supplanted the authority of nurses' professional judgement about their patients' needs for attention.

By the mid-1990s, workload measurement using a hospital's patient classification system had become a central and taken-for-granted technology and its meaning for nursing practice completely naturalized.[24] Patient classification offered cash-strapped hospitals one avenue of relief from the financial pressures being fed into hospitals from provincial governments as federal funding began to dry up beginning in the 1970s.[25] The idea of efficiency that patient classification carries is that not only can nurses actually work faster if they are pressured, but that less nursing work is really needed to adequately care for patients. Technology organized nurses' practice rather crudely, as they adapted to having less time to care for their patients. And that adaptation has taken root.[26] Anyone who has been a patient or has visited a close relative in hospital in recent years knows how much different is a morning on a hospital ward now, compared with the 1981 vignette. Bathing patients, handling food, helping patients walk after surgery, for instance, seem to be 'squeezed in' or overlooked entirely. RNs are busy with other things. This kind of shift both in the content of nursing work, as well as the division of nursing labour, constitutes the lesson nurses learned about their own professional knowledge and judgement – that it could and would be subordinated to the authority of objective measurement.

Patient classification fits into what we have now come to see and call the restructuring of hospital and health care work. Organizing cost savings on the basis of detailed information about care and local accountability for resources began to make paperwork, or its electronic equivalent, a paramount and routine part of health care work. Associated with this work are major expenditures on computers, software, and information management personnel (Krawczyk 1989). These costs are rarely calculated into measurements of hospital efficiency, perhaps because, unlike labour costs, they are 'profits' for suppliers and thus contribute to the economy, as Fuller (1998) would argue. We begin to see how restructuring makes the health care system into a different kind of enterprise from the institution that was established to make health care accessible to Canadian citizens. As Dorothy Smith (1999) has argued, the capacity to organize and control local activities in line with ideas arising elsewhere is a distinctive feature of this stage of capitalism. More than just effective managerial control of hospital resources, the textual processes that addressed the problem of nurse staffing in the 1970s and 1980s should be seen as a forerunner of the technologies that increasingly incorporate health and other professional employees into the ruling apparatus of Canadian society.

Patient classification made it possible for the first time for managerial decisions and organizational priorities to become embedded, through textual processes, in nurses' practice. That effect has continued. Increasingly, centralized coordination of individual hospitals has added to the technical capacity to remedy the 'problem' of nurses' autonomy from managerial control. As nurses are involved in constituting new ways of knowing their work, their own ideas fall in line. In this way, policy decisions made elsewhere in the health care system systematically come to pervade nursing care. The managerial turn in nursing of the 1970s and early 1980s foreshadows the managerial technologies that have been introduced in the years since then. We now fast forward to specific instances of contemporary managerial technologies and related language practices that increasingly dominate nurses' work, and eventually, organize their consciousness.

2 'Three in a Bed': Nurses and Technologies of Bed Utilization

In acute care hospitals there is an inevitable uncertainty about patient admissions, because illness and accidents are unplanned. Emergency admissions account for 50 to 70 per cent of all hospital admissions (CAEP 2001) and cannot be booked in advance. This uncertainty complicates the job of hospital administrators and their new public management strategies that 're-conceiv[e] and, to some extent reorganiz[e], many if not all organizational activities (support and administration as well as production or service) as work processes involving identifiable inputs, outputs and customers' (McCoy 1999: 9). Managing waiting lists[1] and determining who should be admitted next remain big problems for physicians, hospitals, and health authorities. However, a computer program has managed to tame the movement of designated patients into, through, and out of many hospitals, including the hospital studied by Rankin. In this chapter we consider, from the standpoint of nurses, how admission, discharge, and transfer (ADT) software works as a technology of governance within this hospital. Hospitals must account for and manage carefully all the costs of providing hospital care, including the use of buildings and bed capacity – and the latter is where ADT becomes important. Kerr et al. make this case as follows: 'A hospital can only achieve maximum possible efficiency when fixed investments are fully utilized ... If capacity under-utilization exists, fixed costs are higher than necessary and average resource costs of treatment are not being minimized. Therefore, while some degree of spare capacity is essential to meet periods of peak demand ... excessive spare capacity generates inefficiency and needs to be identified' (1999: 640).

Managing bed use and reducing spare capacity become the focus of much of the attention given to effective utilization of the hospital's fixed investments. The area in which the hospital can exercise control is around 'patient turnover,' the hospital production line. The ADT system supports the movement of patients in, through the system, and out of hospital beds, expeditiously, on the basis of information that relates these activities to costs. Inevitably, nurses are involved in these processes, either directly or indirectly, as we shall see. One of the impacts on nursing is in the emphasis placed on discharging patients, as the following observational note suggests. We show that ADT organizes nurses' attention to particular goals and reorganizes their professional judgement and actions in concert with the accounting logic embedded in the technology. As we go on to argue in this chapter and the next, nurses' consciousness is being restructured within a hospital environment that is more and more viewed, understood, and mobilized in relation to the virtual realities of management-oriented information such as that generated through using ADT.

The Discharge of a Postsurgical Patient: An Account of Routine Nursing

The account that follows comes from Janet Rankin's participant observations during the mid-1990s. As a nursing instructor, Janet was updating her clinical experience by working alongside a Registered Nurse (Linda) one morning on a busy medical and surgical ward. Linda's assignment, Janet discovered, was to care for 'all the patients in eight designated beds,' and she was assisted in this work by a Licensed Practical Nurse. The morning tasks revolved around administering medications, assessing patients, getting patients ready for breakfast, assisting them to get washed, making beds, changing dressings and bandages, monitoring intravenous drips, and helping patients to be mobile, in addition to responding to phone calls from families of patients or from physicians and staff in other hospital departments.

Ms Shoulder is one of Linda's assigned patients. An otherwise healthy, middle-aged woman, yesterday she underwent the surgical repair of torn shoulder ligaments (rotator cuff injury). She is to be discharged at 11a.m. Precise discharge arrangements were made well in advance of the surgical procedure during her appointment in the preadmission clinic.

Ms Shoulder has spent an uncomfortable postoperative night. She tells Linda that she slept poorly. This morning, her nursing care focuses on the large shoulder immobilizer she is wearing. The shoulder immobilizer is a type of sling that is worn for six weeks following that particular surgery. It prevents the patient from abducting the shoulder joint (the arm is maintained in a snug position, close to the body; any movement away from the body is to be avoided). Having one arm thus disabled makes it difficult for Ms Shoulder to wash and dress herself. Linda places a chair in the bathroom, provides Ms Shoulder with a towel and washcloth, and tells her to wash what she can and that a nurse will be back later to help her dress. When Linda and Janet return twenty minutes later, Ms Shoulder's face is pale and her skin is clammy. She has managed to wash her hands, face, and crotch but is complaining of severe discomfort in her shoulder and that her stomach is 'queasy.' Linda leaves to get some pain medication, and Janet assists Ms Shoulder back into bed. Linda administers the pain medication (two Tylenol with codeine) and asks Ms Shoulder when her husband will be arriving to take her home. Linda proceeds to do the 'discharge teaching' related to the shoulder immobilizer. Before leaving to attend to her other duties, Linda asks Janet to remove the bulky surgical bandage and replace it with a lighter one. Janet is also to assist Ms Shoulder to dress and be ready for discharge. Getting dressed is a complicated process and takes fifteen minutes. Ms Shoulder requires help putting on her underpants, slacks, shoes, and socks. She is unable to wear her bra and needs help to drape her blouse around her operative shoulder and stretch it across her chest to do up the buttons. She requires help with all the buttons. Once dressed, she appears fatigued and very uncomfortable. She continues to complain of nausea, and at one point Janet assists her into the bathroom, where Ms Shoulder experiences a brief spell of the 'dry heaves.' Janet leaves her resting on her bed and goes to find Linda.

Linda is in the Same-Day Admission Room. There is no bed in this room, and it is not officially part of Linda's assignment. Linda is preparing a newly arrived patient (Ms Leg Wound) to go to the operating room for the surgical procedure of debridement and application of a split thickness skin graft to a large open wound on her leg. Three weeks previously, Ms Leg Wound was hospitalized following a motorcycle accident. She was discharged into a home care program. Her deep leg wound has not responded to the prescribed wound care regimen at home, and now more aggressive surgical intervention is indicated. Ms Leg Wound is in a wheelchair with her injured leg elevated. Linda is going through her chart, checking for a signed surgical consent, looking at laboratory results for particular blood tests, and reading through the physician's orders. Linda is also conducting a short 'preop' interview (last time to eat or drink; last time to urinate, etc.) and ticking these details off on a checklist. She takes the woman's vital signs and assists her out of her clothes and into a hos-

pital gown. The physician's orders include directions to 'compress the wound preoperatively.' Linda unwraps the bandage, assesses the wound, and places a large salt-water compress over it. She will then document a description of both the wound and the treatment. But Janet interrupts Linda to report Ms Shoulder's condition. Linda stops her work with Ms Leg Wound and hurriedly checks Ms Shoulder's chart to see whether she may receive any medications to control her nausea. There is no physician's order authorizing the administration of an antinausea medication, and so Linda, glancing at her watch (and seeing that it is close to 11 o'clock, the assigned discharge time) makes the decision to administer an antacid stating that she 'hopes it will help.' As she does this Ms Shoulder's husband arrives to drive her home. Ms Shoulder is given a prescription for an analgesic and advised to purchase an over-the-counter antinausea drug on the way home. She is given a small cardboard tray in case she vomits in the car. She is then discharged at the required 11:00 a.m. check-out time, looking decidedly unwell.

On the surface, this story about discharging a postoperative patient into the care of her husband is apparently unremarkable. Discharges similar to this happen daily, in hospitals all across Canada. In most hospitals, discharge after rotator-cuff repair happens even sooner after surgery. Indeed, shortly after Janet observed this discharge, the allocated length of stay[2] in this hospital for a patient undergoing a shoulder repair was also shortened, the procedure becoming a 'day care' (ambulatory care) treatment with the patient's discharge slated for the same day as the surgery. But the story about Ms Shoulder has some troubling aspects, including some nursing practice that is unlikely to hold up well to professional scrutiny. We use these observations as an entry point to explore how Linda and Janet's nursing work – not optimal nursing care – happened as it did. We now ask, How it is that two competent and experienced nurses would make these choices about nursing care?

Of possible professional concern would be Linda's breaking of the rule about nurses administering a drug (the antacid) that has not been ordered by a doctor. Linda's administration of an antacid for a patient's complaints of nausea, unrelated to acid reflux disease, did not reflect 'competent application of knowledge' (RNABC 2003) about pain and nausea. More generally, the ad hoc course of action the two nurses followed doesn't exactly satisfy expectations of the code of ethics established by the Canadian Nurses Association that states 'nurses provide care directed first and foremost towards the health and well-being of the client' (CNA 2002: 4). In this situation, nursing actions that demonstrate compliance with professional codes and standards would have seen Linda or Janet phoning the physician to obtain an order for an antinausea medication. After the medication had had time to work, the patient would have been assessed to ensure that both the pain and the antinausea medications were effective. Also, after an uncomfortable night, Ms Shoulder might have been allowed more time to sleep and her breakfast offered later, at which time her discharge teaching could have been given. This course of nursing intervention would have increased Ms Shoulder's ability to be receptive to the important instructions about her shoulder immobilizer, not to mention contributing to her overall comfort and her ability to cope with going home. These choices, optimizing the care of this patient, were not made.

If Linda and Janet's practice is *not* organized by or oriented to professional codes and nursing standards, what *is* its organizing principle or focus? The analysis in this chapter is motivated not to criticize, but to understand how Linda and other nurses working in contemporary hospital settings find themselves unintentionally subverting the standards of their profession. Using the approach of institutional ethnography, our inquiry begins in examining the activities of Nurse Linda, Ms Shoulder, and Ms Leg Wound. That is, we investigate what we see happening and look for clues that we can follow to explicate (the social relations of) how it happens as it does. We notice in the story the way the needs of Ms Shoulder and Ms Leg Wound conflict and recognize that they both are urgent. The urgency that we see relates to several nursing priorities. One is the routine feature of nurses' work – that it is organized to articulate patients to ongoing hospital schedules, such as those of the operating rooms, or to a scheduled discharge. Nurses are trained to finely attune their attention to such schedules and to the associated standard requirements. (Where a patient is not ready for her or his turn in the operating room, there are ensuing consequences for everybody else – all the surgeries for the day will be late, the surgeons will be held up, irritated, and so on; or if Ms Leg Wound goes to the OR without the proper documentation, completed accurately, her surgery may be put off, again creating complications for her and others.) The routine features of the discharge that Janet was instructed to handle as she prepared Ms Shoulder for discharge are also evident. This chapter will have more to say about the consequences of a delay in discharge. But we need to mention here another feature of the urgency of the demands on Nurse Linda's time – both she and Janet are concerned about and try to be responsive to patient comfort and safety. We see how Nurse Linda is caught up in addressing these demands, choosing to interrupt her pressing work with the OR-bound patient.

There appears in Janet's account to be more pressure on Nurse Linda than would be expected in the routine balancing act that is a nurse's everyday work experience. What accounts for this? Is it that she has had an extra patient dropped into her workload? To all outward appearances, Ms Leg Wound is not one of Nurse Linda's assigned patients. But it is not a coincidence that Ms Leg Wound appears now and can demand Nurse Linda's urgent attention. She has been organized to be there. Nurse Linda is not surprised and indeed Janet, too, can now understand why Linda's workload was expressed not as a definite number of patients, but as 'all the patients in eight beds.' We will discover a whole system of organizational texts and people's activity lying behind the arrival of Ms Leg Wound on Linda's medical and surgical ward that tie this admission to the predicted discharge of Ms Shoulder. Here we have an instance of the organization of admissions and discharges that appears to be placing more than one patient 'in a bed.'

The ADT system is instrumental in making the connection between a discharge and a new arrival, and for bringing Ms Leg Wound into the Same-Day Admission Room (and into Nurse Linda's hands). The use of this computerized software program produces an apparently orderly and timely movement of patients into or out of preadmission suites, the emergency room, the admitting department, surgical operating rooms, and beds throughout hospital wards and nursing specialty units. Its use generates the knowledge by which this hospital efficiently manages its 'fixed investments'; but as we shall see, that is not all that happens. Also, as part of the tightened up utilization of fixed assets (namely, hospital space) nursing knowledge is downgraded as a basis for nursing action to the point that we claim that the operation of ADT accomplishes a partial restructuring of nursing practice.

The ADT System: Knowledge for Restructuring

We might describe the ADT system as a patient-tracking system run from a computer on the top floor of the hospital where it is physically removed from the busily peopled settings of the hospital units. But ADT must also be seen as a technology that contributes to the textual (numerically based) monitoring and transformation of the cost-relevant use of hospital beds and other clinical resources. This particular system is a proprietary software program contracted from a company known as Medi-tech. A team of clerical staff, 'patient placement clerks,' work with the system, which requires them to enter demographic patient data into various fields on computer-generated forms. Through other entries in various fields on their computer screens, patient placement clerks keep an up-to-the-minute record of all ongoing hospital admission and discharge activity. The system creates a hospital 'bed map,' which is a bulky document that is printed twice a day. The bed map is organized by hospital units and provides a means of tracking the patients occupying beds throughout the hospital. Bed maps can be printed from computer terminals throughout the hospital and are used by unit clerks and nurses on the wards to keep track of where patients are located. The ADT system also has the capability to produce other documents that are not widely distributed throughout the hospital, for example, the Occupancy Summary by Location form. This lacks any specific patient information, is much less bulky than the bed map, and provides at a quick glance the total number of admitted patients per unit. Other forms generated by the ADT, such as monthly 'inpatient location statistics' and 'total occupancy rates,' are available to departmental administrators and their clerical staff as they gather and monitor data about patient activity in their departments. At this hospital, the ADT system and all of the data it generates are the responsibility of the Director of Performance Improvement and Health Information. The ADT system's 'account' of beds occupied, spare capacity, booked and prospective patients, planned and actual discharges, and so on, enters into and becomes part of a textual reality around which managerial action is coordinated.

The ADT system tracks and locates patients as they are admitted into, transferred among, and discharged from beds. A textual representation of the space availability, and who is assigned to what space, is made and kept updated by the software program. Actually, a patient placement clerk using ADT information, in concert with clerks in the hospital admitting department and the OR booking office, and operating under the authorization of patient services managers, organizes patient arrivals into ward beds. The clerk's work with the ADT system determined Ms Leg Wound's timely arrival on Nurse Linda's nursing unit. It organized which bed she would be assigned to and who might be transferred in order to accommodate her (should Nurse Linda not accomplish Ms Shoulder's discharge on time, for instance).

Assigning patients to beds is no simple undertaking. Beds are chronically in short supply in relation to the number of patients waiting for them. As well, patients cannot be randomly placed into any available bed in the hospital. Patients are assigned to beds based on established protocols related to the nature of their illness, their sex (until recently, about which more is said shortly), and whether they have requested a private room and can be considered 'revenue generating.' The patient placement clerk uses computer-generated bed maps to locate patients and beds and, on occasion, to finesse bed allocation within the virtual reality of the ADT system's bed maps. A patient placement clerk explained this strategy: 'We admit people but we [may] have no beds for them. They come in before the bed is ready for them. So, in the system we create this place called SDAs [Same-Day Admits]. They are fictional rooms.'

Efficient bed utilization is constituted through a textual construction in which 'fictitious' beds apparently expand the hospital's capacity. For instance, Ms Leg Wound was admitted to the hospital, and indeed underwent her surgery, before there was any confirmation that a bed (or a nurse) would be available for her recovery. In the ADT system, the problem of keeping the queued patients in view is solved by the creation of a textual space in which to house them. This capacity to expand fictitiously the number of available beds explains Nurse Linda's comment during an interview when she said wryly, 'You should have been here last week when I had three patients for one bed.' A hospital executive also recognized this phenomenon, calling it '110 per cent utilization.'

The constant overlap of patients shapes the 'speeded up' work processes of nurses who are always, nevertheless, irremediably grounded in the embodied actualities of their daily/nightly work. Patients have bodies and they need real beds. When new patients arrive, they require nursing attention, even if they do not appear in a nurse's assignment. And, besides taking care of the extra bodies, the overlap that the use of fictitious beds creates is consequential for nurses in another way. It is up to nurses to see that the virtual bed into which the new patient is assigned is actually available when the patient needs it. This accounts for Nurse Linda taking 'short-cuts' when caring for Ms Shoulder. It explains why she would have given her discharge instructions when Ms Shoulder was in pain, and it explains why she put aside Ms Shoulder's nausea and discomfort and hurried her out of the hospital. Nurse Linda and her colleagues have learned to adapt their nursing care to the dictates of the hospital's overriding concern about excessive spare bed capacity. This is how the ADT system organizes and even restructures nurses' work.

Placing patients in beds is only one of the uses of the ADT system. Its capacity to represent textually this aspect of the operation of the hospital is important in many other ways. As the patient placement clerk enters information about patients into the computerized ADT program to create bed maps and assign beds, she contributes to the generation of a great deal of statistical information. The number of patients 'in' and 'out' of each inpatient area in the hospital is counted and categorized. Monthly reports generated through the ADT system are circulated to all the patient services managers at the hospital. The monthly reports, known as 'inpatient location statistics,' are organized under the system's headings – 'bed days,' 'patient days,' 'average length of stay,' 'average daily and monthly census,' and 'percentage of occupancy.' Other data generated through the ADT system, and known as 'service statistics,' are collected by the Director of Performance Improvement and Health Information for reporting to the Ministry of Health. Accumulated 'patient days' are broken down into various categories and subcategories. There are (1) 'service' categories (e.g., medicine/general practice; surgery/ear, nose, and throat; medicine/neurology); (2) 'payment' categories (e.g., billable categories such as long-term care and acute care); and (3) categories of 'appropriateness' (e.g., acute care or alternate level of care).[3]

Information generated through the ADT system is also made available to the Canadian Institute of Health Information, and it is this sort of information that the CIHI relies upon when developing case mix groups (CMGs). The product of an administrative classification system used in Canada CMGs group and describe in commensurable form the patients admitted to acute-care hospitals. Modelled after the American diagnosis-related groups (DRGs), CMG systems use data that are routinely generated by hospitals to group together patients who are similar clinically in terms of diagnosis and treatment, and importantly, similar in their consumption of hospital resources. CMGs are then employed to make comparisons of resource use across hospitals with varying mixes of patients. The development of CMGs is thought to produce a sound, up-to-date method for assessing the relative efficiency of hospitals. In the early 1990s the usefulness of case mix groups for determining hospital funding levels was emerging in Manitoba: 'Thus far, Hospital Case Mix Costing is proving to be a highly effective means of assessing hospital efficiency. Ultimately, if analyses in subsequent years continue to support these initial assessments, such data could provide important information with which to adjust global funding' (Shanahan, Brownell, Loyd, and Roos 1993: JS101).

ADT data collection and the various kinds of aggregations made of it render one hospital's costs and use of resources comparable with that of other hospitals. These comparisons (as they affect bed utilization) offer new means of influence over nurses' and physicians' practice. In this regard, a nursing team leader reported how an 'older' surgeon tended to 'hang onto his patients too long' and how this became a problem for her to resolve. She explained how ADT-generated data were useful to her to broach this topic with the offending doctor. She was able to show him how his patients stayed in the hospital longer, on average, than those of his orthopaedic colleagues, and how his practices reflected a wasteful use of the valuable bed resources.[4]

It is the virtual reality of the ADT system that makes it useful for managing beds efficiently. For instance, it is only in a system that creates fictitious beds that the sleight of hand by which people with no beds are counted as inpatients makes 110 per cent bed utilization possible. This careful tracking and overbooking reduces the possibility that any hospital bed is left vacant. However, the fictitious beds of the ADT system create challenges for nurses (such as Janet and Linda) to overcome in that their work is 'on the ground,' with actual beds and actual patients. It is important to recognize that nurses' work in the transformed everyday/everynight world of nursing brings together what actually happens with the virtually generated accounts. In doing so, nurses accomplish in actuality the efficiencies of the rapid turnover.

The ADT system is very much implicated not only in Nurse Linda's work with Ms Shoulder, but also in the work of nurse managers. Interwoven into Nurse Linda's practice are policies and procedures monitored by nurse managers to ensure program efficiencies. New policies must be generated to make the best use of the system's potential. The textual or virtual reality of the ADT system prompts managers to review and revise specific clinical practices. For instance, the decision to designate shoulder surgeries as same-day procedures, reducing the time these patients spend in the hospital, did not arise spontaneously. It was a knowledge-based decision of the sort we refer to as constituting a textual or virtual reality. A patient services director who reflected on how the 'same day' designation was made remembered 'a provincial trend to treat shoulder surgeries as day care.' Knowledge of this trend came to the patient services director in the form of statistics, amassed through the ADT systems of several peer hospitals across British Columbia and reported to the Ministry of Health in the form of monthly statistics. There, relevant comparisons were made across peer hospital groups, and the information was distributed back to the hospitals, thus producing a knowledge base about bed utilization across the province. Prompted by this knowledge about the provincial trend, the patient services director and her management colleagues initiated an examination of their own hospital's practices.

In matters like this, it becomes apparent how the different authority accorded to statistical knowledge overrides a professional's experiential knowledge. One of the patient services managers identified some of the challenges she faced when reassigning shoulder repairs into the ambulatory care program. She explained that 'when shoulders were first being considered for ambulatory care the nurses who were currently caring for these patients on the orthopaedic ward expressed many worries about patient's pain management during that first night at home.' She then added, 'However we knew it could be done, that it was working in other centres; patients at home do well.' What this nursing manager knew was what her statistical information told her.

Her confidence that a patient will 'do well' is based on data collection oriented to statistical outcomes, a major undertaking of health services research.[5] Researchers examine quantifiable measurements such as the number of clinic visits made postoperatively, the time it takes for patients to regain range of movement, and readmission rates of patients who are discharged to their homes on the day of their surgery. Length of stay (LOS) data are then compared with these sorts of (cost relevant) outcomes. All these become indicators of a hospital's performance. ADT systems are relied upon to generate a great deal of the data upon which health services research is based. Mykhalovoskiy identifies how this sort of research 'is highly applied. It does not simply present research findings, but articulates them in terms that seek to organize evidential relations of hospital restructuring and management' (2001: 275). These sorts of evidential claims are different from those of the orthopaedic nurses who were worried about 'how well' patients would do at home following shoulder surgery. For nurses, the patients' experiences of pain and suffering count. While they may be empathetic about patients' pain, another nursing issue is even more important. Before a patient leaves the hospital after surgery, the instructions that the patient is given at the preadmission appointment must be reviewed. Postoperatively, patients must get explicit directions for their own care. Nurses recognize that patients have limitations in what they can hear when they are ill, stressed, or in pain, and that it is nurses' responsibility to ensure that patients (and most often a member of the patient's family) understand their recovery regimens. They know that patients need nurses' time and attention and also that different people need different amounts of instruction. However, none of these nursing concerns get included in the official data gathered to make a decision about how shoulder surgeries are to be accommodated.

One patient services manager identified these differences in ways of knowing when commenting on an initiative she was involved in to make laparoscopic gallbladder surgery an ambulatory procedure. She said, 'I personally am a little reluctant because I think it's a major surgery and I think they can benefit from an overnight stay. However, if I take on that role, that is the nurse coming out in me.' This patient services manager understood that 'the nurse in her' was not properly acquiescent to the authoritative statistical knowledge, and in contrast, her job required her to override these sorts of 'nursing' concerns. She continued, 'We find that nurses do advocate strongly for patients. First of all we have our doctors not wanting to send the patients home, then we have our nurses who can often find reasons why the patients need to stay, frankly some reasonable and some unreasonable, but that they do tend to be protective.'

Such tendencies among doctors and nurses are something to be managed. Authoritative statistical knowledge provides the means through which standards can be developed to compare (virtually) and act on variations among patients themselves (for instance, the levels of pain and nausea such as that experienced by Ms Shoulder) and among professionals ('some reasonable and some unreasonable'). This (nurse) manager concluded by saying, 'I have many years of practice. I am astounded at the changes. It is surprising to me. I have been here for a lot of changes and have been involved in the implementation of change – the pre-admit, and same-day admit procedures where people may have stayed for a month, and now they are going home the day of [surgery]. I am constantly amazed at people's ability, on the whole, to take that on.'

The manager's knowledge about how well patients fare following day-care surgery seems at odds with Janet's experience of discharging a decidedly unwell woman with an emesis basin the morning after a rotator-cuff repair. The statistically generated information also seems at odds with other nurses' experiences of nursing postsurgery patients through the night, before shoulder-repair procedures became part of the ambulatory care program. These nurses explained how, in their experience, the anaesthetic block used to perform the surgery works better in some patients than in others. They noted how some patients experience a great deal of pain and require substantial nursing support, while others do not. Suppressing her own doubts, the manager quoted above remains positive about fulfilling her management responsibility to ensure that patients are not held in the hospital just because nurses or doctors have 'found reasons' to extend their stay. Her role demands that she will monitor and use her information resources to override the 'reasonableness' of the professional judgements being expressed. The new standard for length of stay for shoulder surgery is a case in point. Statistical comparisons such as those being used to justify the change in shoulder surgeries are used to validate that, in fact, patients at home 'do well.' A standard being imposed on all patients makes it difficult to express the sorts of variation among patients that nurses worry about.

Nurse Linda's ad hoc activities that produced Ms Shoulder's 11 o'clock discharge (the antacid, the advice about over-the-counter antinausea drugs, the vomit container to take in the car), examined alongside an administrative decision to categorize the needs and care of patients undergoing shoulder repair as same-day surgeries, provide a particularly compelling illustration of how administrative use of objective health information is employed to make efficiency-oriented decisions and how that reorganizes nursing care. The issue here is how a technology that, in the hands of patient placement clerks and management nurses appears merely to be a useful administrative tool, effectively organizes what nurses can do for patients. The patients, the subjects of nurses' attention, are objectified and become merely 'discharges.' Despite the nurses's qualms, the administrative review of the ADT data from other hospitals did result in an initiative to assign shoulder-surgery patients to the ambulatory care program. This kind of administrative knowledge 'trumps' the local judgement of competent professional caregivers.

The ADT system appears to be a remarkably helpful way of keeping track of where patients are in the hospital in order to reduce excessive spare capacity. We see it as a technology that produces knowledge for managing bed utilization, a feature of the management of efficiency. As the system helps the hospital establish a speedier through-put of patients, the involvement of nurses encourages and even necessitates a restructuring of nurses' work and patient care. The management's version 'of how well we are doing' enters into and displaces nurses' ideas about a patient and how well any individual patient is doing. Nurses' concerns about how well a patient is doing address patients as embodied individuals, the subject of nurses' professional assessment and judgement. The authoritative version reflects objectives related to efficient utilization of resources (reducing spare capacity). Displaced in the latter version are the options about care that nurses would choose and that would better stand up to professional tests of adequacy. Laid over the nursing setting, the objectified knowledge supports processes and procedures that rule the setting. What is known statistically dictates the way that patients will be cared for, subordinating nurses' experience-based worries about patients' variable recovery patterns and different levels of pain and suffering. This theme is repeated, again and again, in analyses that show virtual accounts working better for the managerial agenda than for the agenda of caregiving.

Knowledge Infrastructures Built for Managing Costs

The ADT system builds factual accounts about patients' movements through the hospital – information that stands as a representation of what actually happens as it mediates (or instructs) transformative action. In this section, we suggest how its character as a textual reality is important to its usefulness within the managerial agenda. We have already argued that a textual reality, 'how well we are doing,' should not be mistaken for what actually happens. The ADT information is a built infrastructure. It attends to the placement of patients in beds in a manner that foregrounds efficient bed utilization (costs and accountability) and not, for example, patient preferences. It does this through organizing what will be known in categories that make visible the cost relevance of space so as to support decisions that reduce the possibility that any bed is 'inappropriately' staffed or occupied. With the exception of the actual bed maps, all of the documents generated by the ADT system build utilization statistics through translating the work of nurses and clerks into data that reflect time utilization (such as length of stay data and cumulative transfers) or space utilization (percentage occupancy of beds). Constructing this visibility means that other knowledge related to the use of hospital space drops away. Other ways of knowing what is important are displaced by the more authoritative version carried in the ADT system. For instance, lost are the aspects of patient placement to which nurses might give priority, such as using space flexibly to enhance the comfort of patients. Nurses who Rankin interviewed described how difficult it was for them to arrange to have dying patients moved into private rooms or to have patients who were having trouble sleeping moved out of rooms where a roommate snored loudly. They were critical of the amount of authority that the patient placement clerk held in relation to decisions to move patients throughout the hospital. They felt it constrained their own ability to accommodate patient care.

The ADT-inspired transformation of the hospital will have variable outcomes for differently located groups of people. ADT information fits with and advances actions framed in relation to efficiency. It does not have the same internal relation to nursing goals and actions. Managers are 'instructed' in various ways by the ADT system's statistical information. In one case, a new policy about 'same sex' rooms was generated to capitalize on the faster through-put of surgical patients. Speeding up the treatment of surgical patients through preadmission and same-day admission procedures creates bottlenecks, with many more patients present than available beds. This combines with the inherent unpredictability of patients requiring emergency admissions, who also end up 'lining up' in the emergency department waiting for available beds. Almost always, there is backlog of patients waiting to be accommodated. Customary rules about same-sex accommodations became a drag on the most efficient use of bed capacity – that ADT-based placement otherwise made possible. The placement clerks would have to handle the problem through complicated 'transfers.' A patient placement clerk described the challenges she encountered daily at 4 p.m. This was the 'cut-off time' when further discharges were unlikely, and she could reasonably predict that all the patients in the hospital would be staying the night. She had to find everybody a bed, and eventually she would run out of appropriately sexed beds. Creating fictitious beds was no longer a solution because patients would be physically waiting in various holding areas of the hospital. Transferring patients among rooms would become the only way to 'find beds.' The clerk gave an example of the 'just awful' work this entailed:

> I mean some of our moves are just awful. ([Say that]) we have two four-bed male rooms, and each one has an empty bed in it. But we need three

female beds. So you have two empty male beds but no empty female beds. So then you empty a semiprivate room, move two of the guys from the four-bed rooms into the semi, then you move the third guy from the four-bed room into the fourth bed in the other male room, and now you have four empty beds you can put ladies in. I mean they can even get more complicated than that ... sometimes you're moving people all over the place just to get the right combination of same-sex beds.

She was describing the complexity involved in transferring patients virtually from one space to another, as she used her bed map to 'juggle' and 'squeeze' patients in, to maximize the bed resources within sex-segregated restrictions. For the patient placement clerk the work of transferring patients to find beds is a complex computer puzzle. Through manoeuvring patients on her bed maps, she is able to make highly pressured decisions about where patients can be placed in the hospital. But her account of 'awful moves' is nothing compared with the embodied work of nurses who actually move beds, patients, and their belongings. When the instruction comes from the ADT clerk, nurses begin pushing the beds, gathering belongings from bedside lockers, informing the receiving nurses about the condition and needs of the patients being moved, and gathering and moving the appropriate records, medications, equipment, and so forth.

Using the cumulative ADT-generated statistics of 'awful moves,' managers, too, can 'see' the labour involved in transferring patients. For them, costs and efficiencies are paramount. Transferring patients from room to room is yet another cost to try to reduce. When patients are moved from one bed to another it involves not only the patient placement clerks and nurses, but also ward clerks, housekeeping staff, medical records personnel, dietary clerks, and so forth. Records must be adjusted and extra work done to accommodate patient transfers. For this reason, the patient placement clerk explained, patients who are in four-bed wards or semiprivate rooms are seldom moved to accommodate mere preferences (for instance, a preference to be placed by the window or nearer the bathroom). Rather, transferring a patient from one bed to another is most often reserved as a tactic to 'find beds' (or to accommodate a 'revenue generating' patient who has requested a private room and can be categorized as a 'paying private'). Transfers are carefully monitored. According to the patient placement clerk, when the ADT system showed a continual increase in the number of patient transfers – the 'awful moves' – managerial attention was brought to bear on this issue. The resulting change in policy was unisex accommodations. Unisex realizes significant organizational efficiency by ensuring that no bed remains empty owing to it being treated as inappropriate by virtue of the patient's sex. One manager interviewed about the new policy viewed unisex accommodations as a way of 'letting go of outmoded rules and moving into the new millennium.'

It seems clear that ADT information helps hospital managers consider how to facilitate the efficient use of resources. In that light, the new unisex policy is successful in alleviating an apparently wasteful use of hospital space and of hospital workers' labour. What remains invisible within the picture created through the ADT system is the impact on patients. When the textual representation is substituted for knowledge of the local experiences, managers miss patients' responses. It is likely that the new work that is undertaken in order to function within the new systems is also overlooked. We learned about the discomfort of mixed-sex accommodations from Mary, a single woman of sixty-seven who was experiencing unstable angina and spent sixteen days on a heart monitor awaiting a coronary angiogram. Mary was accommodated in a room with three men, with whom she shared a bathroom. She found this upsetting. She felt it to be an assault to her modesty. She said that she kept the curtains pulled (and pinned) around her bed all the time. Trying to maintain her privacy increased her isolation and her sense of vulnerability, as she adjusted to sharing sleeping, toilet, and bathing space with men. Such issues become a mere 'preference' that hospitals cannot accommodate.

Even if managers were sympathetic to patient responses, individual managers do not have the privilege of using their discretion about such things. The ADT information is part of detailed information about hospital activities that is made available to managers with the expectation that it will be used to improve hospital performance. Performance here means adequate care with minimized expenditures (Shanahan, Brownell, and Roos 1999). ADT-generated statistical data, aggregated and fed back to the hospital managers, have already been used by government funders to establish 'provincial averages' and 'benchmarks' that hospitals have to live up to. Subsequent reports will compare them with like hospitals and like regions, and hospital administrators live in an ever-tightening loop of performance of efficiency in relation to other hospitals.[6]

Hospital managers are harnessed to improving hospital performance, not only through their job descriptions and upper management expectations, but also through the version of reality that the information provides. For instance, the patient services director's knowledge about how 'well' patients do at home following shoulder surgery is factual. It is based on statistics. Standard statistical measurements offer the kind of description of hospital performance and health care delivery that produces unassailable accounts. Another director interviewed explained how having only just returned from holidays he had decided to take the 'period statistics' home to review them. Embedded in his talk about his use of statistics is the reliance he places upon them for his decisions: 'At any given time we can pull the statistics. Actually, we're not doing very well right now. We've started to vary a little bit with our hips and knees, probably by a day or two here and there. We have to get better at that.' When he says, while looking at the statistics, 'we have to get better at that,' he is referring to his managerial responsibilities, organized through the facts generated by the computerized systems of counting, including ADT. The information-based work of these directors, and the accounts their work generates, produce the hospital efficiencies that are the imperative of cost containment demanded in health care reform. This is specialized work and it constructs a particular perspective. Pulling sheaves of paper from his briefcase the patient services director explained how he works in this textual medium, and how he is accountable to the ADT-generated data:

> We need these statistics for a couple of reasons. We [report] those ones that the ministry insists on and I need some purely to do my work. I use them as backup for proposals. I guess every second day you get involved with discussions with other hospitals in comparative talks. You get at the table in budget discussions or whatever, and you can talk statistics at people. We can say, 'Okay yes, well we do 280 joint replacements a year, so we do need more money in our Joint Program.' Utilization and length of stay are big issues with the region. They say, 'Look here, what's happening here? You're not utilizing well' ... and certainly, in our discussions with the ministry, in order to receive any extra funding, for the Joint Program for instance, they talk about length of stay and utilization a lot.

He uses his statistically generated knowledge when interacting and negotiating with people from the Ministry of Health, for whom 'utilization and length of stay are big issues.' As a manager it is his job to initiate strategies to address the problem of patients and practitioners who 'vary a little bit,' with the result that patients stay in the hospital 'a day or two longer' than their allocated five days. It is his responsibility to organize professional practitioners and hospital employees to direct their work towards standardized length of stay for patients. For him, the ADT data provide the facts of efficiency, towards which his everyday work is directed. In our analysis, efficiency is shown to be a virtual reality, a construct of particular categories chosen for how they can make commensurable patients, treatments, beds, length of stay, utilization, and so on.

Information about the movement of patients through cost-relevant spaces is used to maximize the efficient use of resources not only in the day-to-day admission and discharge or sex-segregation practices being managed locally, but it also informs decisions being made by bureaucrats and public administrators far removed from the actual sites of patient care. In British Columbia, certain funding decisions are made based on a hospital's performance, calculated on the basis of the ADT data. In health care reform and hospital restructuring, hospital administrators, regional health authority administrators, and bureaucrats at the Ministry of Health all make use of the ADT-generated data to make decisions such as the closure of hospital beds, the closure of hospital wards, or the closure of entire hospitals. Major redesign plans are generated by regional authorities. For example, one B.C. health authority cut nine beds from a local community's hospital, and when a great outcry ensued, relied upon calculations gathered through the ADT data to explain the proposed changes. Although it was true that service demands were high in that community (higher than in some comparable hospitals), length of stay was also 'significantly higher [at 7.8 days] than the 4.8 average days per case for similar conditions in comparable hospitals.' Better utilization management was expected to make the nine-bed closure able to be absorbed 'without compromising patient care' (Petrie 2003: 3–4).

When patient placement clerks use ADT to distribute patients, the patients enter (and later, the system requires them to leave) a nurses' work purview. In drawing attention to how statistical information collected in this system informs policy decisions that are to improve hospital performance, especially the hospital's efficiency, we have shown how useful it is to have this kind of cost-relevant information. We want to put that together with our ethnographic analysis and reflect on the different standpoints represented. Our analysis draws attention to what is not known, at least not authoritatively, about the impact on individuals of policies that put efficiency in the forefront. At the level of managerial decision-making, clinical relevancies about how patients are to be accommodated, or which patients require overnight care, fall out of sight. We showed Nurse Linda scurrying about making room for incoming patients, her nursing care being aligned with and constructing, in actuality, the hospital that is modelled in the ADT system's virtual reality. In these same activities, Nurse Linda's work is also being aligned with policy – the reform and restructuring agenda. She and her nursing colleagues work to the demands made on them.

We end this chapter on a troubling note. The accounting logic being appealed to in the restructure and redesign of health care systems propels continuous 'improvement' in efficiency. The whole health care enterprise is being thought of as a virtual reality whose efficiency and productivity can be endlessly enhanced. A hospital president described an instance, in 1997, when the regional hospital he administered received funding for '673 acute inpatient days [i.e., funded beds] per 1,000 population.' He explained how, statistically, this translated into two overnight beds per thousand people in the region. Then his hospital's same-day admission program and improved ambulatory care procedures generated improvements in utilization, and the data sent to ministry officials via the ADT system reflected this. That year, the ministry readjusted the 'benchmark targets' for 'acute inpatient days,' reducing the funding that would be made available from two to one-and-one-half beds per thousand population. A continuous ratcheting up of productivity expectations occurs. This accelerates the demands that are fed into nursing.[7] Nurse Linda's increased pace of work, her ad hoc nursing, and her suppression of nursing values are what it takes to coordinate the work on the ground with the virtual reality of the information-based technologies. Together they accomplish the goal of a restructured hospital and, at least for the immediate present, demonstrate 'efficiency.'

3 Doing the Right Thing at the Right Time: Adjusting the Mindset of Nurses

It is midmorning on a busy urological unit and Registered Nurse Trudy Mills, returning to work after four days off, finds Mr Jones slated for discharge into the care of his wife. Mr Jones is an elderly patient who is recovering from major surgery – a radical retropubic prostatectomy – for prostate cancer. Trudy recognizes from his patient record that it is his 'day seven' meaning that his treatment is or should be completed; Mr Jones either is discharged now or reclassified to non-acute status on the urological ward Trudy had nursed Mr Jones before her days off and remembers that his post-surgical care was complicated by his mild confusion, his fear, and, especially at night, his tendency to become combative when approached. Now, four days later, with his stitches out and his urinary catheter removed, he seems better. Trudy assists him into his underwear, a pair of comfortable elastic-waisted 'track pants,' and a warm sweater, noting at the same time that his incisions are clean and well healed and that he can move easily. She gathers up his slippers, housecoat, and cane and gently assists him into a chair to wait for his wife. Moments later, Sara Haynes, the Licensed Practical Nurse with whom Trudy is working, notes that Mr Jones has been incontinent of urine, and his track pants are soiled. She helps him into the bathroom where she washes him and assists him into dry pyjamas, adding an incontinence brief underneath the pyjamas. But now Mr Jones gets irritated, and it takes all of Sara's skill to get him to cooperate to return to his chair. Outside the room, Trudy is at her medications cart, and Sara reports what has happened as she goes to get a plastic bag for the soiled pants that Mr Jones will take home with him. When Sara comments that 'This old guy is pretty cranky.' Trudy frowns thoughtfully and replies, 'Yes, I think his wife is going to have her hands full.'

This vignette holds traces of several restructuring strategies that are entering nurses' work. Two of them are analysed in this chapter to show that virtual realities generated within and integral to these strategies supplant nurses' knowledge and eventually displace their judgement. Unlike the admissions, discharge, and transfer (ADT) system discussed in Chapter 2, the restructuring technologies we analyse here target clinical practice. The first is a clinical pathway. Mr Jones was at 'day seven' of his clinical pathway, the day scheduled for discharge. Second, the vignette hints at case-typing – a technology that kicks in when a patient such as Mr Jones is finished his acute treatment process and yet for some reason cannot be discharged.

The similarity between the clinical pathway and case-typing is that they are both text-mediated technologies, and like the ADT system, they advance the efficient utilization of hospital resources. Use of a clinical pathway advances hospital efficiency by standardizing and streamlining the treatment regimens for patients with certain diagnoses. The clinical pathway holds nurses and other caregivers to a predetermined treatment schedule that has as an endpoint the patient's timely discharge. Case-typing relies on nurses to identify patients who, according to standard criteria, are inappropriately occupying acute-care beds. The case-type designation 'alternate level of care' (ALC) that we discuss later in this chapter initiates a textual tracking process that generates information feedback to the hospital about the costs incurred for such patients. The designation also triggers a differentiated and reduced nursing regimen for these patients. We argue that the virtual realities that are generated in these two separate technologies are new forms of knowledge that subordinate nursing knowledge and thereby restructure nurses' judgement and action. This analysis begins to show how nurses develop an organizational consciousness that is aligned with restructuring priorities. Not only, as seen in Chapter 2, do nurses make choices about nursing to conform with new tightened schedules, but in this chapter we show nurses revising their own judgement in line with managerial knowledge. This is a subtle advancement of accountability logic into the mindset of nurses.

'On the Seventh Day ...' – the Use of Clinical Pathways

The importance of 'day seven' to Nurses Trudy and Sara is that their patient, Mr Jones, has been processed on schedule through the standardized treatment as set out in the clinical pathway. On day seven, he is to be discharged. Use of a clinical pathway tidies up what can otherwise be very divergent treatment practices. Technologies of this sort are expected to 'improve patient outcomes, meet standards and facilitate easy tracking of a patient's progress' (Windle 1994: 80F). Building upon evidence-based medicine, clinical pathways are the documentary form of a 'best practice' or what Timmermans and Berg (2003: 25) call a procedural standard. Implemented in a treatment unit, clinical pathways establish, direct, and record (for monitoring variances) key interventions by all clinical staff occurring at timed intervals throughout a patient's hospitalization. Pathways have been developed for a wide variety of medical diagnoses and surgical procedures. At a glance, a caregiver can see 'whether or not the patient is following the defined standard pathway without incident or if there are significant variances' (Windle 1994: 80K). The discovery of a variance would call for specific attention; otherwise, the treatment is standard, as the text indicates. To be effective as an efficiency tool, the clinical pathway must not only be developed in line with scientifically validated 'best practices' but it must also be used systematically. Since its use reorganizes the practice of all of the people who are involved in caring for the patient, special efforts may be needed to gain the necessary compliance of caregivers. We had an opportunity to see how nurses in the hospital that was studied were participating in the new technology.

Tracking the Development and Implementation of a Clinical Pathway

While Rankin was conducting observations on an orthopaedic ward, the nursing unit manager was charged with developing and implementing a clinical pathway. An excerpt of the pathway for a patient undergoing total hip replacement surgery (hip arthroplasty) is shown in Figure 3.1.

Managers in the hospital studied had decided to institute a clinical pathway on this unit because the average length of stay for hip and knee surgeries surpassed the benchmark that the provincial government had established. According to a Ministry of Health report the hospital was 'remiss in employing effective utilization management efforts in order to ensure the residents have reasonable access to health care services' (Regional Hospital, Financial Management and Operational Assessment – Review Team Report 1997). Implementing the pathway was supposed to remedy the hospital's (i.e., its clinical staff's) perceived inefficiency in performing its public function. This conclusion about the hospital's inefficiency had been drawn from aggregated health information that compared the productivity of peer-grouped hospitals.

Figure 3.1: Clinical Pathway

TOTAL HIP REPLACEMENT CARE PATHWAY					
O.R. DAY-POST OP Date:_____	**DAY 1** Date:_____	**DAY 2**	**DAY 3**	**DAY 4**	**DAY 5** Date:_____
1.TEACHING/DISCHARGE PLANNING - D B & C - Foot and ankle exercises - Turn with an abductor pillow/other - PCA/pain control	- D B & C - Reinforce hip precautions - Review pain control --> transition to oral analgesic - Bed exercises - Activity progress	•••••	•••••	•••••	- Review precautions; equipment, home exercises - Referrals arranged
2. ACTIVITY - Turn q2-3h in bed with assist, Abductor pillow in situ - D B & C - Foot and ankle exercises	- Turn q2-3h in bed with Abductor pillow - Bed exercises - Stand with walker	•••••	•••••	•••••	- Final Review with O.T. - Physio final review exercises and gait - Meet at vehicle to check transfer method
3. ADL's: - Independent as able - Major assist with bath and diet	- Major assist with bath and diet	•••••	•••••	•••••	
4. DIET: - sips --> clear fluids	- Clear fluids --> general	•••••	•••••	•••••	- General
5. MEDICATIONS/IV THERAPY: - Maintain IV - PCA - I.M. pain med - Indocid Suppository - Anti-emetic - IV antibiotics X 24h - Transfuse blood as per orders - Anticoagulant therapy	- Cap IV if Hgb > 90 - D/C antibiotics - Begin oral analgesic overlap with PCA - Daily coumadin administration - Personal meds - Indocid Suppository	•••••	•••••	•••••	- Oral analgesic - Coumadin - Personal meds - Iron supplement
6. ASSESSMENT /THERAPY - Post-op head --> toe - Neurosensory check q1h X 2; if stable q4h - V.S. q1h X 2; q4H - Monitor and empty drain q4h - Fluid balance - O2 per nasal prongs - Monitor urine output and empty q12h - Pain scale - Check dressing: reinforce X 1 - Place bed in Trendelenburg position	- Neurosensory checks q4h - V.S. q4H - D/C drain - Fluid balance - Monitor urine output and empty q12h - Check dressing: operative leg edema; assess DVT - Skin integrity assess q shift with bath or turns - Chest and abdomen assessment - Trendelenburg bed when patient at rest	•••••	•••••	•••••	- Neurosensory check q shift - V.S. O.D. pm - Operative leg edema; assess DVT - Skin integrity q shift - B.M. assessment O.D. - Trendelenburg bed - Leave clean, dry incisions open to air
7. TESTS:	- Hgb - INR	•••••	•••••	•••••	- INR

Nursing became, within the hospital's schema of counting and comparing surgical productivity and benchmarking, a de facto problem to be resolved by better management. For the treatment of patients undergoing arthroplasty to be speeded up, the treatment schedule was to be directed by a clinical pathway. Nurses would have to work differently from how they had learned to nurse in school and how they had honed their skills through experience. The clinical pathway establishes an efficiency-oriented treatment process that handles this 'nursing problem.' Vested in texts – forms, charts, and so forth – clinical pathways coordinate the efforts of nurses and allied health professionals across time and space, ensuring that their activities are indeed standardized.

Clinical pathways establish new nursing activities and alter nurses' recording practices. We see this reflected in the minutes of one meeting between nurse managers and the clinical pathway implementation group. The group had been discussing whether or not the pathways text could replace, altogether, nurses' existing charting protocols. The minutes read: 'In any case, it was felt that the charting would have to be left as it is but we could use the care map as a *mind-set and objective* for the staff, and as a score card. It was decided that the [clinical pathway] would go into the chart where the relevant discipline, be it Nursing, Physio or OT will circle the item that a patient has not met for that day if appropriate' (emphasis added).

Note that the focus of the implementation group is on adjusting nurses' mindset. Placed in the patient chart where nurses are already charting, the text of the clinical pathway adds a simple 'circling' of any item that falls outside its established course: that would be a variance. This is an apparently small change in charting practice. Yet once nurses learn to address the expectations for their involvement in each of the seven categories of treatment, and as they adopt the mindset of the predetermined therapeutic goalposts and timely discharge, they become the pathway's agents. Adopting the mindset and undertaking the activities, nurses' work along with the work of other involved practitioners accomplishes the standardized length of stay. Nurses take on the task of monitoring the patient's progress, even of monitoring their colleagues' attention to variances. The clinical pathway technology organizes nurses to see and accept *as a nursing concern* the goal of five-day hospitalization for joint replacement.

Nurses' active involvement in the operation of a clinical pathway is crucial to its success as an efficiency device. Nurses are drawn into and enact a particular relation. Here the crucial coordinating work is textually mediated. As text, a clinical pathway is a material form of a social relation that hooks nurses into the ruling practice of hospital restructuring. It is simply 'text' until nurses (and, in this case, other members of the orthopaedic treatment team) activate it. The problem that managers have to solve, referred to above as nurses' inefficiency, really is a problem of gaining nurses' active compliance in the managerial goals of early discharge. Nurses have to 'forget' their previous ways of working, including their commitments to responding to patients as individuals, and follow the pathway's instructions; thus, the aim is altering nurses' mindset. The mindset represented in the clinical pathway is 'the primacy of early discharge' authorized by the scientific evidence standing behind it. The clinical pathway process is the methodology that accomplishes the early discharge: 'It [the clinical pathway] achieves the coordination of all the team members so that each person knows what needs to be done and when ... it means you don't have to wait around to get an order to get patients going. Nurses can start to generate discharges on admission' (Interview, Patient Services Manager).

Gaining nurses' active compliance with this restructuring device requires some effort on the part of nurse leaders. Nurses must be taught and required to practice differently. Nursing's front-line leaders (in this hospital, called the 'unit managers')[1] are enrolled in activities that orient nurses to the primacy of the discharge. In the case of this clinical pathway, the unit manager conducted a library search, consulted with other hospitals that had already adopted a clinical pathway (a large tertiary care centre in Ontario and a smaller centre in Washington state), and carefully negotiated the 'orders' directed in the pathway with the local orthopaedic surgeons. This is work that orients nurses to the pathway to ensure its regulatory effects. In the orthopaedic ward, the implementation group used what they called 'whistle-stop' sessions and other in-service classes to teach nurses about clinical pathways.

The clinical pathway provides a means of managerial influence over work that previously was regulated professionally. According to the manager interviewed above, the pathway organizes the multidisciplinary team to know 'what needs to be done and when.' It directs nurses to 'start to generate discharges on admission' and by focusing on daily 'targets' established for each preplanned day of hospitalization, nurses accomplish the restructuring goal of greater efficiency. But besides taking over direction of nursing care, the technology also makes certain aspects of nurses' work visible to greater scrutiny and open to correction. Nurses' recording – their circling of variances in the clinical pathways text – produces a system for organizational surveillance. Earlier, we saw the managers discussing the potential for the arthroplasty pathway to be used as a 'score-card.' The minutes of the implementation team's meetings reveal the subtle form of regulation that is being inserted into nurses' practices. Presumably, professionals and treatment units will be compared according to scores achieved through their discharging success. Local adaptations and permutations of clinical pathway technology are being implemented in hospitals all across Canada. Windle's (1994) description of the implementation of a clinical pathway in a postanaesthetic recovery room explains how pathways work to regulate nurses in that setting. In hospitals such as the one Windle describes, the surveillance methods may be an integral component of the pathway technology. She found variances being documented in terms of 'delays' that were categorized specifically in relation to 'the patient,' 'the system' or 'the caregiver' (1994: 80K). Thus, in the recovery room Windle studied, each delay could be attributed precisely to a cause and even to the culpable professional member. In the orthopaedic unit where we analysed the implementation of the clinical pathway, the surveillance and accountability systems were less formally specified, but the technology still worked to regulate nurses' practice.

An interview with the nursing unit manager who had led the pathways project revealed how use of the clinical pathway had evolved at her hospital. Insufficient funding for the project meant that despite having staff 'circle the item that a patient had not met for that day,' variances were no longer being monitored. The manager was frustrated that her vision for the project had not been fully realized. Nonetheless, she noted that since implementation of the clinical pathway 'the ward has been much more consistent with our five-day discharges.' Use of the pathway, nested in a set of authorized standard doctors' orders and with ongoing coaching and mentoring of nurses, accomplished the discharge targets without explicit monitoring of variances. The daily practices of doctors and nurses had changed. Having adopted the mindset of the five-day discharge, nurses themselves took up the responsibility of keeping patients 'on track.'

Tracking How the Pathway 'Works': Organizational Consciousness

The work of nurses such as Sara and Trudy, whose activities we described in the opening of this chapter, has become aligned to the efficiency mandate. Interviews suggest how this was accomplished at the cost of the exercise of nurses' own judgement about caring for their patients. The case of Mr Jones is one such instance. Trudy described in more detail the knowledge she drew upon that guided her practice with the patient on the morning of his discharge. She described how, in her previous night shifts, she had nursed Mr Jones during his early postoperative period. He had been confused, calling noisily for help, and kicking out when approached by the nursing staff. Trudy explained how she had reported her patient's night-time confusion to the nurse coming on duty, prior to leaving for her days off. Trudy then described how, upon returning to duty, she was once again assigned the care of this patient: 'Anyway, I come back to work and according to all the paperwork it's day seven and he's ready to go home. So you wait for his wife to come in, because you know she is going to have her hands full, you need to explain to her what to watch for.'

Trudy now had to mediate the care of her patient through the requirements of the clinical pathway. She recognized that even though Mr Jones was 'ready to go home' he was still recovering and would need substantial nursing assistance from his wife. Trudy's professional work includes teaching and support for both the patient and especially for the home caregiver, whose successful participation makes the hospital's whole efficiency project possible. Trudy had to explain things to this elderly couple about pain management, how to look after the surgical incision, and the need to avoid straining during a bowel movement, and she had to give instructions for Mr Jones to avoid heavy lifting. She might also have explained about the not uncommon experience of postoperative urinary incontinence and taught Mr Jones how to perform perineal exercises. She continued her story explaining: 'His wife arrives and I introduce myself and I'm trying to figure out who she has already talked to, and I'm trying to slow down so that I can give her all this information in a way so that she won't be too overwhelmed. I am rushing though – through the discharge instructions, the prescriptions, his bowel meds, and stuff. So I'm talking to her, explaining about his incontinence and telling her where she can buy Attends [adult diapers].'

It is relevant to what happens that Trudy's own available time is a limited resource. She described how she was aware that she was 'rushing' – to find out what the patient's wife has been told by other nurses and the surgeon. She engaged in the work of priorizing – to discover what still needed explaining. This work requires sensitivity. Trudy had to be attentive to the capacities of the people she was teaching. She said that she reminded herself to 'slow down' because the wife was overwhelmed. As the discharge session progressed Trudy explained how, despite her teaching interventions, Mrs Jones was signalling serious concerns about her ability to cope with the care of her ill husband. About Mrs Jones, Trudy said: 'She gets all welled up and tells me that he has been hard for her manage at home even before his surgery, and she starts to talk to me about how he's been ... and even though home support has been put in, she's still in over her head.'

Here is where the efficiency squeeze interferes with the nursing care. Even though she had assessed that Mrs Jones was 'in over her head' Trudy's options for what she can do are limited. She is working in a situation organized according to managerial, not clinical interests. The ruling concern is to clear the patient's bed. Being part of this organized setting affected Trudy's own thinking, her mindset. Her acceptance of the organizational need to accomplish this discharge overruled any nursing judgements that might disrupt the organization. She explained: 'But it's already too late, you see. The bed's already booked, we are already looking for beds for five same-days [patients admitted that morning and currently undergoing surgery] and so far we only have two, this old guy and one other, so already we're three short. And you know the pressure is on.'

The pressure Trudy was under to accomplish this discharge was evident in what she said about the 'line-up' of patients waiting for beds. Five beds were needed; and so far, only two had been identified as becoming available, even though at least one of the 'available' beds (Mr Jones's) was still occupied. On this day, like many others, there was a serious negative balance of beds for patients who had already been admitted and were undergoing surgery. To delay the discharge of this confused elderly patient would have created significant problems for the organization.

A social organization external to her nursing work influenced Trudy's thinking and her approach to her patient. She saw that this couple was not really ready to cope with the man's care. Whatever interventions Trudy's professional education and experience may have suggested, her talk revealed that what she decided to do was organized by 'bed pressures.' The institutional agenda for routine and timely discharge intervenes. Trudy explained how she responded to these pressures: 'So you talk to the Team Leader to see if you can get more home follow-up on this guy, but he's got to go, it's day seven. I mean there's just no way. I can't hang onto him because his wife got teary. So I mean, you just kinda kindly bundle them out the door and keep your fingers crossed that home care will catch up with them, and then you start looking after the next one. And let's face it, it might feel like hell, but that's not our job. I mean, it might not look like it's very caring, but it's just not efficient use of resources to hang onto this patient for another night just because his wife is having trouble coping. There are all those other patients waiting for surgeries to think about.'

The practical problems related to holding this nurse's worksite together are evident. Despite the fact that 'according to all the paperwork' this patient was ready for discharge, the nurse identified patient issues that do not show up in the virtual reality. As with Linda's work with Ms Shoulder (described in Chapter 2), Nurse Trudy, too, was faced with developing an ad hoc plan. In this case, advice to stop at the drugstore on the way home to purchase adult diapers was accompanied by an attempt to organize more home support.

The contradictions Trudy faced in dealing with the Joneses are evident when she expressed how her work 'might feel like hell' and how it 'might not look very caring.' Her description of her practice revealed a 'moment of recognition that something chafes' (Campbell and Gregor 2002: 48). It is exactly moments such as these – in the everyday / everynight practices of front-line nurses – that strategies of restructuring must subordinate. The nurses' mindset as developed through clinical pathways ensures an *organizationally correct* course of action. In restructured hospitals nurses become knowledgeable actors in the 'efficient use of resources.' Nurses learn that diverting a discharge to address a wife's tears and concerns about coping is *not* their job. The nurses' job is to think about 'all those other patients waiting for surgery.'

Trudy responded, as she had to, to an organized and systematic process for moving patients into, through, and out of the hospital. The 'paperwork' she referred to is the clue being explicated here, when Trudy explained, 'Anyway, I come back to work and according to all the paperwork it's day seven ... but it's too late, he's got to go, it's day seven.' The fact that this patient was 'day seven' authorized how Trudy knew how to proceed in that situation. Knowledge about what 'day seven' means trumped what else she knew about this patient – it overruled her own doubts about her discharge activities. Despite the fact that Trudy described how 'it might feel like hell,' she subordinated her other ways of knowing about how to carry out her nursing work. She rationalized her actions through her knowledge of bed pressures and waiting lists and constructed her understanding about competent nursing practice within the scarcity and rationing practices of contemporary health care reform and hospital restructuring.

These data about a nurse discharging a patient are analytically useful in demonstrating what Dorothy Smith calls the transformation of (a nurse's) organizational consciousness: 'Progressively over the last hundred years a system of organizational consciousness has been produced, constructing "knowledge, judgement and will" in a textual mode and transposing what were formerly individual judgements, hunches, guesses, and so on, into formulae for analysing data or making assessments. Such practices render organizational judgement, feedback, information, or coordination into objectified textual rather than subjective processes' (1990b: 213–14).

We have shown how Nurse Trudy was conscious of the efficient use of beds and of her overriding professional responsibility in relation to that goal. Her practice was being organized in the way that she 'knows' it through the accounting logic embedded in the clinical pathway's discharge scheduling, tied as it is to hospital data collection, benchmarking, hospital comparisons, and ultimately, finances.

Nurses are organized to compress caring into smaller spaces. They are also learning how to download costs for supplies and equipment into the home sphere and to make use of family members as surrogate nurses. Trudy, working with an elderly couple who faced multiple challenges related to cancer, surgery, incontinence, cognitive changes, and so forth, explained how she 'just kinda kindly bundled them out the door.' She relied on the somewhat tenuous plans for home care, trusting that something had been organized ('keeping her fingers crossed'). She understood and justified this version of nursing practice through her knowledge about 'day seven' and the 'efficient use of resources.'

Text-based technologies such as the clinical pathways being described here are designed to govern practitioners' knowing and acting. They systematically and quietly insert the relevance of 'counting' and 'benchmark targets' into nurses' everyday/everynight activities. Patients with cardiac illness, patients undergoing surgeries, and even patients experiencing mental health illness are grouped and categorized to determine 'optimum' (efficient) lengths of hospital stay that can be defended as evidence based and quality assured. In accordance with this 'medico-administrative' data (Mykhalovskiy 2001), discharge targets are developed and strategies are employed to organize and focus nurses' work around a planned discharge time and date. The regulating features of the clinical pathway are designed to merge compatibly with the physical organization of patients entering and leaving hospital beds that pulls nurses along with it. In Chapter 2 we displayed how, by following the standardized discharge protocol for her patient who had undergone shoulder surgery, Nurse Linda was contributing to the efficient running of the ward. Until Ms Shoulder (among others) physically left the hospital, her presence constituted a constriction in the rolling out (in actuality) of the virtual order of the bed map. Disrupting this order not only disadvantages another patient but creates trouble for the unit manager, the surgeon, the operating room staff, the bed utilization clerk, the admission staff, and so forth.

The development of the clinical pathway tools creates a nursing framework through which nurses can uncritically bend and fold their traditional professional interests in nursing their patients (Ms Shoulder's nausea and Mr Jones's confusion and incontinence) *into* their new professional responsibilities for restructuring care. Despite knowing that their patients would benefit from more nursing care, Nurses Linda and Trudy both subordinated their professional impulse and responded instead to more compelling knowledge. 'According to all the paperwork' these patients had fulfilled predefined criteria for discharge. This is the moment when managerial knowledge and authority overwhelms a nurse's traditional professional training about adequate nursing intervention. In the next section we examine case-typing, a managerial technology for categorizing patients in relation to how acute their medical problems are, and see how it also comes to dominate nurses' thinking and actions.

Alternate Level of Care: 'These are patients who really shouldn't be here'

In the vignette about Mr Jones we were introduced to his wife, the family caregiver, into whose hands he was being discharged. The nurses understood that Mrs Jones carried the weight of the early discharge that the clinical pathway established. Nurse Trudy recognized the fragility of this link; it may not hold. What if Mr Jones had not had a wife? Or what if his wife could not have been persuaded to take on the complicated demands of her husband's postoperative convalescence? For these situations, another managerial strategy is available. Case-typing is a technology that hospitals use in an attempt to identify and to circumvent some of the costs of having non-acute patients occupying expensive acute-care beds.

As a managerial technology, case-typing is made possible by the routine collection of special health information. One such case-typing technology is known in the study hospital as ALC, an acronym for alternate level of care. The ALC technology is used to screen and redesignate patients in acute care hospitals in relation to their unsuitability (from an administrative perspective) to be there. During her participant observations in hospitals, Janet Rankin first encountered the term ALC in nurses' talk during shift-change reporting. She noticed how, in nurses' card indexes and worksheets, ALC appeared as the patient's diagnosis. At first, being unfamiliar with this acronym, Janet had assumed it was a new medical diagnostic abbreviation or acronym, such as ALS (amyotrophic lateral sclerosis) or CHF (congestive heart failure). Upon inquiry, the nurses explained that ALC means that patients so designated 'really shouldn't be here.' This section of the chapter describes how ALC data are generated, reported, and aggregated, producing a virtual reality upon which important decisions about hospital operations are made. We argue here that the ALC-produced virtual reality does more than improve the cost effectiveness of hospital resources. Introduced into the nursing lexicon, ALC becomes a powerful regulator of nursing work, and another way of adjusting a nurse's professional mindset about the nursing resources that should be devoted to hospitalized patients.

How Alternate Level of Care Works

Unlike the established sorts of clinical diagnoses from the International Classification of Diseases, or the North American Nursing Diagnosis (NANDA) categories, ALC is a category developed for and relevant to managing hospital resources. Despite the ALC designation not being designed for clinical decision-making, nurses and physicians are the primary actors in the ALC designation process. For the most part, it is nurses who do the work to identify patients who meet the ALC criteria as they have been established by the Canadian Institute of Health Information (CIHI 1997). It is nurses who prepare the ALC forms and who undertake responsibility for securing a physician's signature that formalizes the ALC designation.

Also known as 'inappropriate days' or 'lag days,' ALC is a term used to identify patients who although judged to be ready for discharge or transfer are 'inappropriately' occupying an acute care-bed. In CIHI literature an ALC patient is defined as 'a patient who no longer requires acute care but continues to occupy a bed for any reason' (CIHI 1997).

Our research shows that the inclusion of ALC as a diagnosis within a hospital ward's working texts offers nurses a way of talking about and knowing their patients that is distinctively differently from how they are accustomed to thinking about them. Three separate texts are involved in this technology: the doctors' board, the ALC designation form, and the nurses' worksheet.

'The doctor's board' is a wooden clipboard to which a form is attached (see Figure 3.2). The form lists the names, diagnoses, and location of each patient who is currently occupying a bed on the ward. We shall see that it is exactly the same photocopied form that the nurses use as their 'worksheet'; however, when attached to the doctors' board, the far right column is for communicating patient issues that require a doctor's attention. As an organizational text, it is an informal working one that is used, then discarded and replaced every day. This text is part of the ongoing conversation between doctors and nurses that constitutes their coordinated effort of caring for patients. Attending physicians and surgeons look at the doctors' board when they visit episodically. Rankin found it posted at the ward's main desk. Nurses make notations on the doctors' board to bring their concerns about patients to a doctor's attention. In the case of ALC, nurses' comments prompt the doctor to consider whether a particular patient might be so designated. On the board, the prompt usually appears as the cryptic query: '?ALC.'

In contrast to the informal textual domain of the doctors' board, the ALC designation form is part of a bureaucratic textual domain. Its use initiates a variety of text-mediated actions.

The ALC designation form has a tick-box format with no space for narrative elaboration (see Figure 3.3). It comes with a set of instructions for its use and as such offers clues regarding the organizational discourses it enters. Statements in this text assert that information will 'assist with discharge planning' and will be used for 'data collection.' The form outlines a protocol for identifying patients who fit the ALC criteria. A doctor must authorize the designation and tick-boxes are provided to indicate particular 'barriers to discharge,' for example, 'family caregiver unavailable,' 'awaiting test or procedure,' or 'long-term care bed unavailable.'

Despite the authority for ALC designation resting with the physician, it is nurses who do much of the work that it entails. All levels of nurses screen the patient population for potential ALC candidates, consulting with one another and sharing their judgements via notes in

Figure 3.2: Attention Doctor Form

Attention Doctor

Room	Patient Name	Diagnosis	Physician	Comments
301-1	70 Rite, Brian	Chest Pain Rule Out M I	Spencer	Please reorder hydromorphone 6mg SR capbid
301-2	67 Soley, Derek	LLL Pneumonia	Yue	IV iscut. Patient is a difficult start. May we leave it out?
302-1	72 Wigmore Otto	COPD	Yue	Phone sister re test results please.
302-2	87 Schapoks Bryan	Urosepsis	Yam	? ALC
303	86 Nagra, Jagtar	ALC	Clements	

Figure 3.3: ALC Designation Form

DEFINITION OF ALTERNATE LEVEL OF CARE (ALC)
An Alternate Level of Care patient is a patient who has finished the <u>acute care phase</u> of his/her treatment.

(The following information is required to assist with Discharge Planning and for the purposes of data collection)

☐   **ALC: On Admission**   Reason: _____

☐   **ALC: Waiting Placement** – type of placement requested:

      Extended Care ☐   Intermediate Care ☐   Rehab. Facility ☐

☐   **ALC: Other** _____

☐   **Discharge Plan in Place   Y ☐   N ☐**

☐   **Barriers to discharge:**

COMMUNITY	HOSPITAL	PATIENT/FAMILY

Waiting LTC
  Assessment
Long Term Care Bed
Unavailable
Home Nursing
Unavailable
Waiting Home Care
Assessment
Home Support
Unavailable
Other
_____
	Waiting Test/Proc
	  Specify
	Delay Test Results
	 ☐ Lab ☐ X-ray
	Other
	_____
	_____
		Refuse LTC
		Respite
		Family Caregiver
		Unavailable
		Other
		_____
		_____

(A patient is classified as ALC when the patient's physician indicates that the patient no longer requires acute care)

☐   **ALC: Designation Date:** _____
                                    Day   Month   Year

_____
Physician Signature

the doctors' board. Nurses' preparation of the ALC text for the doctor's use includes stamping it with the designated patient's name, birth date, hospital number, and physician's name. This clerical work may fall to the nurse manager, whose responsibility for generating acceptable statistics finds her actively procuring the physician's necessary signature. As part of getting the form completed, nurse managers will also frequently have to explain to physicians the particular 'barrier to discharge' that applies to the patient in question.

Completed ALC designation forms travel from the ward to the hospital records department, where the information is entered into a computerized database. The standard format of the ALC text is designed to funnel local information into statistics generated by the Canadian Institute of Health Information. And aggregated data on this class of patient make their way back into the hospital where they inform decisions at an organizational level, as we describe later in the chapter. At the unit or ward level, ALC designation is already actively influencing nurses' knowledge and their work with patients. Once a patient is officially designated ALC the designation is documented under the 'diagnosis' column of nurses' worksheets, alerting nurses to the designation.

The nurses' worksheet, like the doctor's board, is a member of an informal textual domain. The nurses' worksheet is exactly the same as the photocopied form attached to the doctor's board, however, this version of the form is used differently. Each nurse carries her own worksheet. It was this tool that Rankin saw nurses using during her shift-change observations noted in this book's introductory vignette. The worksheet is a pocket-tool providing nurses with a quick reference about the care and reporting responsibilities that they hold for assigned patients. As with the doctor's board, the right-hand column is empty, and in this space nurses enter details that they consider relevant to their day's work.

Inquiry into how nurses use the worksheet shows how they address themselves to and take up a diagnosis listed on it. One RN explained, 'I write down all the stuff from change of shift report and then refer to it during the day.' The worksheet is filled with the specialized language of nursing (and medicine), and a diagnosis calls up for nurses their knowledge of the nursing action that they are expected to take. For instance, one nurse used yellow highlighting on her worksheet to identify three patients in her care who were diagnosed with a 'C. *difficile*' infection, a particularly contagious bowel bacteria that requires nurses to use special isolation precautions. The diagnosis cues the nurse to take up this diagnosis knowledgeably, delivering the care that ensures that it is worked on competently during her shift. Besides being an aide-memoire concerning care to be given, this nurse also used the worksheet to prepare her report to the nurse to whom she would turn over her patients: 'I sort of fill in the blanks and then before I go in to make report for the next nurses coming on duty, I go through the sheet and make notes about anything that is important, like when I gave that guy his last shot, or who has a low blood sugar, or if I am worried about a wound or something.'

From interviews it became apparent that various levels of nursing staff take up the ALC designation differently. Responses from licensed practical nurses, registered nurses, and nurse unit managers indicate what the ALC designation means to their different work responsibilities. For instance, LPNs do not interpret ALC in its institutional sense. We found no traces of any of the uses organizationally established for the ALC designation in the LPNs' talk about the 'diagnosis' of ALC on their worksheets. LPNs seem unaware of its institutional purposes such as the 'development of criteria to use as a yardstick for measurement' (Dick and Bruce 1994: 98) or 'to enhance Provincial and National Comparisons' and 'to provide valuable information for planning purposes' (CIHI 1997: 2).

In the hospital where Rankin observed nurses working with ALC on their worksheets, a protocol was developed to reduce the minimal required standard for nursing notations to be entered into patients' records. In addition, patients designated ALC are not required to have their blood pressure, temperature, and pulse monitored on a daily basis. Pragmatically in this way, the ALC designation directs the work that nurses are required to do for the patients. When asked whether the 'diagnosis' of ALC (as it appears on the worksheet) actually influenced the care she gave, one LPN responded: 'It doesn't really make any difference when [my patients] are designated ALC. *It's great that we don't have to do the vital signs and chart,* but really they still need the same kind of care. They need bathing, they need to eat, they need lots of bowel and bladder care ... many of them are incontinent or else need frequent toileting. I mean the work doesn't really change' (emphasis added).

It is LPNs who have been organizationally positioned to initiate the ALC designation; they identify candidates and prompt the registered nurses and the nurse unit managers to seek this designation from the physicians. For the most part, it is the LPNs' work to measure and record the vital signs for all patients. Thus, their workload is reduced and made more manageable under the ALC designation. This may have been their motivation as Rankin observed them enthusiastically recruiting patients into the category.

A somewhat different understanding emerges from asking RNs how the designation of ALC on their worksheets relates to the care that they give. RNs also talked about the time pressures on their work, but in addition, their talk was inflected with traces of gerontology as a specialized body of nursing knowledge. Woven into their understanding of the needs of ALC patients was a conception that 'the frail elderly' require different approaches and services than are available in the acute-care setting. This is how one nurse put it:

> I find having a lot of ALCs can be difficult. They have different needs than the acute patients. They often take a lot of time because they are old, and most of them are really dependent. I mean, that's why they can't go home because they need all this help. We should be working towards keeping them as independent as possible, but that takes time ... I do use a different mindset with these people. I feel sorry for them. There's not a lot we can do for them here. Sometimes they stay for weeks, and you can just watch them slipping away. They lose their confidence. We watch them getting increasingly withdrawn ... I try to make sure they get up in the chair and have some sort of stimulation. I mean we should be dressing them and everything, but it's difficult. We're just not set up for that sort of thing here.

This talk reflects the professional and theoretical interests of the RNs in the life-span development of the frail elderly that include concepts such as 'quality of life.' The interview data revealed that nurses' work with ALC patients is complex and difficult. RNs frequently commented on the *extra time* that long-term, stable, but physically dependent patients require. About their ALC patients, they said, 'They're slow'; 'they're often confused'; 'sometimes they are combative'; 'they are heavy physically'; 'they take a long time to feed'; 'they have a hard time swallowing their pills'; 'many of them are incontinent or require frequent toileting'; 'you know, you can't rush these folks.' Additionally, the RN's comments reflected how nurses *plan and order* the care of ALC patients: 'often they just have to wait'; 'they're not as sick as the other patients and if I have to decide I have to look after the sick ones first';

'they're the stable ones'; 'I focus on the assessments and treatments of the acute patients first.' Nurses expect that patients in acute care will get better and move on. The patients who stabilize, but who are unable to move on, provide a distinct set of challenges for the nurses. Although nurses know about the skilled and delicate acts of caring for frail, cognitively and physically disabled elderly people, these RNs nevertheless failed to be convinced that ALC-designated patients actually deserved their care.

Their talk reflected the assumption that the acute-care setting *is* inappropriate for ALC-designated patients. It appears that the nurses interviewed had incorporated into their own thinking a particular understanding of what should happen in hospital units, an understanding that is being inculcated through the use of clinical pathways and other strategies of efficient management. Patients' needs, they seemed to be saying, should match what is offered, instead of the other way around. Recovery times, for instance, are standardized without regard to age differentials. This organizational thinking has been naturalized. It becomes common sense, and unhooked from any obvious connection in these nurses' talk to the efficient use of fiscal resources or of staff productivity – which is the CIHI agenda for the ALC designation.

Nurse managers understand ALC as a method of influencing 'bed utilization.' Their talk was infused with concerns about the budgetary constraints they were facing and the need to 'do more, or at least the same, with less.' Talking about how the ALC case designation was useful to her as a means of monitoring the bed utilization on her ward, one nurse manager was very interested in knowing how many patients within her ward population 'really need to be here' and getting 'a handle on the types of patients who are taking up the beds.' Organizationally positioned to take responsibility for the costs of running their nursing units, the nurse managers most frequently interact with physicians in interpreting the ALC criteria, reviewing discharge plans, and encouraging physicians to either discharge patients or to designate them ALC.

Although only physicians have the authority to officially enact the ALC designation, for a variety of reasons, they are the professionals who have the least invested in this work. It is nurse managers' responsibility to liaise with the physicians who, because of their private billing practices, have long been exempt from certain managerial relationships with the hospital. Nurse managers, who are employees of the hospital, undertake responsibility for completion of the ALC texts that record, organize, and monitor the 'medical decision to be made by the attending physician or authorized hospital designate to determine when a patient no longer requires acute care services' (CIHI 1997: 2). This nursing management work is a key link in restructuring.

Once it is officially authorized by the attending physician, the ALC designation form initiates a series of textual responses as it enters into the bureaucratic modes of action for which it is designed. This initiates a 'distinctive circularity' (Smith 1990b: 97), as ALC becomes enacted within the textual realities of health care administration. The special code given to an ALC-designated patient is used each time information about that patient is entered into the hospital ADT database. Through the ADT database the hospital accrues local statistical data related to the numbers of ALC patients present in the hospital population. Information related to ALC patients is tallied monthly, and along with other ADT-generated statistics, it is regularly reported to the Ministry of Health and ultimately to CIHI. At CIHI, 'hospital summaries' are compiled and distributed back to all comparable 'peer' hospitals.

Summaries contain statistical comparisons among hospitals, such as 'percentage ALC days' relative to 'total patient days.' ALC-designated patients appear in these summaries as total cases, care-types, resource-intensity weights, and a percentage of hospital weighted cases. All these data are relevant for costing, comparing, and making managerial decisions about the efficient use of hospital facilities and resources.[2] The virtual reality produced by ALC case-typing technology is about the appropriate use of labour resources rather than, as in ADT technology, the efficient use of available space. As an administrative database, ALC information can be used to make the difficult decisions of hospital restructuring that restrict the type of nursing and medical care to which certain patients may have access. ALC foregrounds the hospital's business-oriented practices of calculating the efficient use of labour resources and it backgrounds other issues, for instance, ones that emerge in the care of frail elderly people whose healing and recovery vary from the established norm, who cannot be discharged, and who for various reasons continue to occupy hospital beds.

As seen already, case-typing has particular meaning for nurses and nursing care. Classed as 'inappropriate,' ALC-designated patients' requirements for nursing care stand outside and beyond what nurses in acute care should understand as reasonable. The construction of the ALC virtual reality inserts administrative interests into nursing care decisions. It is our contention that case-typing through the ALC technology and related on-the-job training develop in nurses an organi-zational consciousness centred in organizational restructuring. For instance, the bulletin entitled 'Understanding Alternate Level of Care' (CIHI 1997), posted on the ward where Rankin interviewed nurses about ALC, summarized an 'ALC Information Session held in April of 1997.' It hints at how nurses' views are being brought into line with others that are managerial: 'Twenty-three participants representing uti-lization management, admitting, health records, social services, finan-cial planning and nursing were in attendance. The attached document is a summary of the questions discussed at this session' (1997: 1).

The questions discussed included: 'Why is it important to identify ALC days?' 'Who identifies ALC?' 'When is ALC documented on the patient record?' 'Does ALC status mean that the patient must begin to pay for treatment?' 'Does ALC designation affect the Resource Inten-sity Weights (RIWs)?' 'How does the Health Ministry use ALC data?' (1997). The questions and answers assume that everybody in the hos-pital has the same interests and that those interests are managerial. The practices being explained (and that appear rational in the restructured environment) begin to reorganize nurses' professional commitments. These commitments, for instance, as they are outlined in the Canadian Nurses' Association code of ethics, learned in nursing school, and expressed in nurses' work during a shift of duty, would be organized around the details of individual patients' experiences. However, they are being reoriented by the practices surrounding ALC, where nurses' clinical thinking is supplanted by a cost orientation. The effects go far beyond the managerial organization of efficient utilization of re-sources. Methodically inserted into the local sites of nursing practice, this kind of training about ALC technology becomes integral to the new 'reformed' framework of nursing action used by nurses to justify difficult decisions about who is an appropriate recipient of their care and who 'deserves' the finite resource of nurses' time. Applying this framework of cost relevance to actual people through ALC-designa-tion processes requires nurses to think of people in *its* terms. We observed nurses referring to patients through this lens (appropriate vs inappropriate, important vs less important needs, deserving vs unde-serving candidates for care, or 'bed blockers'). The cost-relevant frame-work enters into how nurses make their own decisions about who gets their time and attention, and who doesn't. The circle is closed.

The use of ALC as a diagnostic term marks a distinct change from patient diagnosis grounded in traditional medical or nursing science.

When nurses take up ALC as a diagnosis, they are inserting manage-rial concepts and values into their clinical judgments. Nurses are learn-ing that it is the exercise of good professional judgement to allow ALC patients to fall to the bottom of their priority list within the limited resource of their time. Nurses come to understand that these patients 'really shouldn't be here.' Thus, nurses learn how to work within a hierarchy of legitimacy for health care that is constituted through the *particular* knowledge generated for managing the hospital. Health information technologies such as ADT, clinical pathways, and ALC inserted into nurses' direct care of patients shift the locus of control over that care. The information collected and aggregated through the use of these technologies produces the virtual reality that authorizes administrative decisions to take priority over the clinical expertise of nurses and physicians.

There is a fine line in hospital restructuring between efforts that coordinate health care activities in the most effective and efficient man-ner possible and intrusion into the clinical practice in the name of the common good. Much debate centres on related issues – the ethics of medical decision-making, how the capacity to pay might or should mediate the practicalities of treatment, how to decide when treatment becomes too costly, and so on. These are serious issues of public policy. Our focus is much more modest – to demonstrate how knowing a health care setting in a particular way makes it over, transforming it into a manageable terrain, and in so doing, how it affects what actually happens in ways that may be invisible and unexpected.

More and more, at every level of health care, people are making decisions based on information abstracted from the everyday world and constructed within accounting logics. Even small debates such as when a patient is sent home from hospital come under the influence of the accounting logic. Decisions that seem to be about efficiency turn out to have other implications – including ethics, by another name. Inserted at the site of nursing care, the abstract logic of accounting dis-places nurses' awareness about the ethics ingrained in their reformed work. Abstracted aggregates of numbers on length of stay, variances in treatments, 'ALC days,' and so forth, also deprive health care debates (e.g., about the rationing of health care to certain sorts of patients) of a certain specificity. Dissenting opinions are easily quieted by referring to statistics.

To make health care more efficient and effective is the expected goal of restructuring. We have been concerned in Chapters 2 and 3 to demonstrate the effects on our nursing informants of restructuring to accomplish these ends. We have shown that managerial relevances have been displacing the traditional relevances of nurses' caregiving. Nursing judgments are affected by reframing and reconstituting what nurses 'know' through the use of a variety of sophisticated managerial technologies. But the successful restructuring of nursing knowledge requires a complex orchestration of the social relations of nurses' work. Nurses are professionals who hold both individual and collective values about what constitutes proper nursing care. The restructuring of nurses' knowledge does not automatically follow hospital restructuring as night follows day. Some nurses resist the new textual incursions into their practices, finding that the textual work itself drops to the bottom of their priorities during a shift of duty. To teach nurses their 'new' knowledge, and to ensure that nurses participate competently in activities that allow various new institutional manoeuvres to be made, additional managerial and professional strategies have had to be devised. This is an issue that we take up in the following chapter where we describe a group of nurses who speak out about their workplace concerns. The activities of these women guided our investigation into the reformed work of head nurses, who are located differently from staff nurses with respect to the reach and accomplishments of these technologies.

4 Managing Resistance to Restructuring: The Ruling Work of Nursing Leaders

In previous chapters we have shown managerial technologies working up aspects of hospital activities into cost-relevant information used for, among other things, coordinating nurses' activities. These technologies do not directly control nurses' actions but, rather, individual nurses activate managerial technologies 'knowledgeably' (thus, the attempts to influence nurses' 'mindset'). As nurses adopt the technologies and the concomitant mindset, a managerial perspective emerges as dominant. But the terrain in which this happens is contested. It is true that nurses often recognize the utility of the new technologies for solving problems that they encounter in pressured workplaces. Yet in some situations the organizational goal of efficiency may chafe, and nurses may try to counter it. They may resist the new coordination of their work, when they think it imposes unacceptable demands on them and erodes nursing care.

The official sanctioning of management technologies does not by itself ensure their use; monitoring and enforcement is needed to achieve the desired level of involvement on the part of nurses. Carrying out this responsibility is a corps of nurse leaders who bring to it new techniques. In this chapter we describe the reformed work of front-line nurse leaders in restructured hospitals and explicate how a changing conception of 'clinical leadership' and new responsibilities for rationing resources alter the work traditionally done by head nurses. Moving away from their primary interests as clinicians, teachers, and local coordinators of nursing care, the new front-line nurse leaders learn to apply text-based methods of managing nurses and nursing. Our analytic interest lies in demonstrating how these are practices that rule.

Nurses United for Change: What Resistance May Look Like

In the course of her ethnographic fieldwork, Janet Rankin occasionally met with a group of nurses who were unhappy about what they saw as compromised nursing care. Rankin's notes about the actions that this group of nurses undertook form the entry point for the analysis in this chapter. We can see in them the transformation of nursing leadership that is part of the restructuring of hospitals, nursing, and patient care.

Eight nurses from a general surgical ward of a regional hospital have gathered in the living room of a suburban home to voice their concerns about patient care in their hospital. Their talk circles round the loss of a valued head nurse. It has been about a year since the job description for head nurses was changed and at that time their head nurse resigned. A new front-line nurse leader, called 'Clinical Coordinator,' was appointed. She is unpopular and these nurses believe her to be incompetent. They see that she is not providing the clinical leadership or the support for patient care that they are used to. Each nurse has a story to tell that supports these views. One nurse relates an incident about a patient who suffered cardiac arrest moments after being admitted to the ward from the Emergency Department. Upon review of the emergency room records she noted severely compromised blood oxygen levels. This nurse believes that this patient was unstable at the time of transfer and that the transfer of critically ill patients from emergency is a recurring problem. She had asked the Clinical Coordinator to raise these concerns with the Clinical Coordinator of the emergency room, but feels that her concerns have been dismissed. Another nurse recounts the distress of a recently hired nurse who had made a serious blood transfusion error. The nurse telling this story believes that the Clinical Coordinator was partly to blame, not only in the actual error but also for the outcome for the new nurse (she is considering leaving her job). The Clinical Coordinator is criticized for not taking responsibility for her part in the error and also for not being sufficiently supportive around the disciplining of the new nurse. Yet another story finds the Clinical Coordinator culpable in a situation where the nurses had been having trouble getting a doctor to re-evaluate a head-injured patient. And so the stories go. As the nurses express their frustration, the discussion gets more and more passionate. They agree to meet again to try to figure out what to do, under the name they have given themselves: 'Nurses United for Change' or abbreviated, simply 'NUC.'

The original impetus for NUC meetings was criticism of the new clinical coordinator. But eventually discussions covered a range of problems occurring within their nursing environment, including experiences with quality assurance. The nurses had become alarmed at the frequency of lapses in patient care and were determined to make a difference. They took advantage of the formal incident-reporting process that in this hospital was called quality assurance documentation. The QA reporting process was strict; nurses had to complete and submit the required document within 24 hours of the identified incident. Depending on the complexity of what had happened, the forms took about thirty minutes to complete. To finish them in time, sometimes nurses missed coffee or meal breaks or had to stay late following their 12-hour shift. That was a significant cost to these nurses who, like nurses everywhere, would be anxious to go off-duty. So, the QA process itself was a disincentive for nurses to use this method of addressing their concerns. But these nurses persevered even when, disappointingly, they got little or no response except when, on two occasions, they were publicly berated by physicians for reporting incidents that had involved them.

The nurses used the QA process to report any kind of incident that they thought undermined their nursing care. They had submitted several QA forms that documented instances of severe skin blisters caused by a new product that was being used in orthopaedic surgery. One nurse even brought her camera from home, took photographs of the blistering, and attached them to her QA form. The nurses reported several occasions when they had been unable to locate the on-call anaesthetist when they needed to consult him about patient-controlled analgesia. Several of the documented incidents related to medications that had been incorrectly dispensed by the pharmacy.

At the same time the nurses were launching their rigorous QA initiative, an external nursing review team was appointed by the Ministry of Health to assess 'nursing operations' at the NUC hospital. The purpose of the review was to 'briefly review and compare acute care nursing staffing levels at [named hospital] with other hospitals in Peer Group 2 to assess the impact of restructuring on the nursing department.' The reviewers were to use 'workload financial data and scheduled hours' to 'evaluate each acute care cost centre within the Nursing Department, both for comparisons over time and comparisons across peer hospitals' (External Nursing Review, June 1996). NUC saw the appointment of an external nursing review team as a way to get their concerns on the record and, although their nursing managers attempted to deter them, NUC submitted a report to and met with the reviewers to discuss many of the incidents documented on the QA forms. Despite these efforts, the nurses were frustrated to discover that none of their issues appeared in the review's executive summary. The nurses were puzzled as to how the reviewers could write that 'overall the consultants were impressed with the quality of care provided and the effectiveness of resource utilization throughout the department.' NUC believed their concerns had not been taken seriously. The only finding that alluded to any troubles read 'some units within the hospital are having more adjustment problems than others' (External Nursing Review, 1996). It seems that the nursing review, generated from textual data such as workload records and financial accounts, could not integrate the nurses' firsthand accounts. Apparently too, the QA forms that the nurses had assiduously completed were not sufficient to offset the reviewers' claim of an impressive quality of care.

Increasingly disturbed by what they saw happening in their work and the apparent inattention that their reports were receiving, the NUC group decided to take their criticisms directly to the nursing management. A meeting was organized and the nurses wrote up a summary of their concerns for inclusion in the meeting's agenda. Together, they gave careful consideration to how to phrase their concerns. However, choosing what they already understood to be the proper form in which to speak about their problems had an effect that we now recognize. We argue here that working within the organizational framework, and adopting what they thought would be the correct language recast the nurses' observations about what was wrong. The NUC nurses attempted to formulate their message in coherence with the hospital's quality assurance process, shifting its ground so that it could be responded to within the managerial technology, drawing attention away from what had actually happened. A review of the account that they prepared for the meeting shows this happening. The NUC agenda item read:

Quality Assurance Issues: This is an issue of nurses feeling disrespected, not supported and not listened to. It is an issue of professionalism. Nurses need to feel they will not be victimized, marginalized or dismissed when they identify and document their practice issues. Specifically with QA forms, nurses need to understand the process the form enters, they need to hear back [when they document concerns] and they need to feel that nursing management supports the staff nurse standpoint in QA issues. Nurses need to feel supported when they identify QA issues that involve physicians or other departments. Currently there is an utter lack of response; on the rare occasion when a response has been elicited, it is threatening and inflammatory. (May 1996)

Notice that in this statement of what the NUC wanted managers to discuss, the nurses have made the QA forms and process its focus, submerging their own workplace problems. The minutes of that meeting, excerpted below, reveal that nursing managers responded in exactly that way. They took the opportunity to explain the QA process – as if the nurses didn't know it. A nursing manager described how complaints or incidents are to be categorized and handled. Whereas the minutes of the meeting suggest, to us, that the nurses had been finding the process of making QA reports anxiety-provoking,[1] the nursing manager reassured the nurses that the QA process was trustworthy.

We speculate on what may have happened when the concerned nurses identified certain conditions of the nursing unit to be potentially unsafe and asked for them to be addressed and remedied. The next step may have been to subject the nurse who made the report to an investigation; her own practices in the situation may have been questioned. The credibility of her report may have been questioned. She may have felt that she was being listed as a 'trouble-maker' or a 'whistle-blower.' However, the nursing managers insisted that the nurses would be mistaken to think that using an incident report to identify who made the error was 'meant to be punitive'; rather it was the best and most systematic way for managers to follow up and ensure quality of care. The minutes read:

Lorraine [the manager] discussed the QA process:

QAs related to med. errors/falls – Incident reports are not meant to be punitive but rather a means to track problems and ensure quality care. The QA goes to the CC/CN [clinical coordinator / charge nurse] who notes the recommendations, if any. This needs to be completed within 24 hours. The QA then goes to the PCM [patient care manager] who checks if the audit is complete. Patterns are looked for and stats are tracked.

Doctor-related QAs – The RN documents for the CC to follow up; then it goes to the PCM for follow-up; then it's acted on by the chief of staff; this leads to a response and trends to be noted. Dr follow-up can take 6 weeks to 3 months.

QA memos related to burned mattresses and pillows – Again, need to be completed within 24 hours. Maintenance [Dept.] has been made aware, new bed lights have been evaluated; results went to Maintenance; new lights have been ordered from Capital Equipment.

(Minutes, Joint Management Meeting, May 1996)

It seems apparent from these minutes that QA reports are now part of a numerical accounting of problems that occur in wards. They can be integrated with other reports (e.g., of audits) to create statistics and show patterns and trends and that have who knows what uses, but are automatically followed by managers as 'proper procedure.' The minutes suggest that the managers at this meeting were satisfied with the processes in place for reporting these or similar problems. The managers were doing their job by reiterating the requirements for how nurses were to complete the QA reporting, accurately and in a timely fashion. Where they could, the managers explained the action being taken in response to the nurses' reports; where apparently nothing had come of nurses' reports, they explained the lengthy bureaucratic processes that would be engaged. But how would this meeting have helped the nurses whose complaints were really about lapses in adequate nursing care – complaints that they attributed to things outside their own control? The serious issues that the nurses had been raising in their own conversations have disappeared into and been satisfied by the discussion of the QA process.

While it may have satisfied the nursing managers, the meeting did not satisfy the nurses involved. But it did have an effect. Rankin observed that their talk at their regular NUC meetings shifted. At first they had discussed actual events and actual troubles – about heavy workloads, lack of clinical leadership and support in specific cases, the unavailability of doctors to respond to nurses' concerns about patients, faulty equipment, and actual troubles experienced with other hospital departments. These are the types of problems that in the past would have routinely claimed the attention of a head nurse and that these nurses saw as the clinical coordinator's responsibility. Those in the NUC group were frustrated that their clinical coordinator seemed to have no interest in solving their problems. After what they felt was the dead ending of their involvement in the QA process, NUC resorted more and more to impugning personal characteristics of their nursing leaders.

The NUC meetings became consumed by the nurses' attempts to explain the 'utter lack of response' that their actions were garnering. They spoke less about the actual patient care incidents that they were finding so troubling. Instead, the meetings began to focus on concerns about a 'lack of respect,' 'lack of consultation,' and 'not being listened to.' They understood themselves to be 'professionals' and that their professional concerns were not being addressed. In their attempts to be taken seriously as professionals they became more militant, and they went public with these criticisms. They submitted a written report to their local health authority and gave it to a journalist who was sympathetic to their cause. Nonetheless, their many stories of patient care being jeopardized dropped out of sight. Their public action attracted the attention of the hospital president (executive director) who asked them to meet with him (he also met separately with the nursing managers). He concluded that 'the staff/management culture at the hospital was severely damaged' (Internal Memo, Executive Director, 1998). A private consulting company was contracted to work with the nurses and their managers to 'reach agreement on the kind of climate (behaviours) that will be supportive of raising, addressing and solving problems collaboratively' (Internal Memo, Consulting Group, 1998). After that, both NUC and their managers began to focus on their interpersonal relationships and what was called the 'toxic organizational culture.' Framing the problems this way diverted attention away from the actual conditions of the nurses' work – their concerns about patients and their worries about the competence of their new team leader.

Clearly, our observations of the NUC activities do not tell the whole story. And, of course, in institutional ethnography, we do not expect them to do so. As Dorothy Smith (2001) reminds us, institutional ethnography expands observational methods by its interest in understanding the use of texts of all sorts – the activation of which constitutes organization. Our analytic focus remains on the social organization of these nurses' experience. The account that we have included here helps us identify the nature of the inquiry we are undertaking and offers some entry points for it. The Nurses United for Change were incensed about many things going on at work that, taken together, seemed to be interfering not just with good working relations, but with patient care. They saw something that was happening that worried them. Our notes have not reproduced that 'something,' nor is it enough to use either the nurses' accounts or our reconstruction of them as explanation. Rather, we take the standpoint of these nurses as our starting point to explore what they and others thought of as a 'toxic organizational culture.' In this construction of the problem, 'people, their doings and the everyday production of the existence of an organization or institutional order' (Smith 2001: 172) have disappeared. We want to learn how the particular circumstances of these nurses' work lives, characterized as 'toxic,' had been organized. For instance, was this series of unhappy events related to, and even organized by, other changes in this hospital? Because the new text-based technologies that restructure hospital organization are always played out in the settings where nurses work, nurses are caught up in them, and as we have already argued, nurses are often responsible for their successful implementation. This puts nurses and their work into the centre of the work environment that is being restructured. The NUC were particularly critical of working with their new clinical coordinator, and so in this chapter's analysis, we begin there, learning how nurses at this level in the organization, the front-line nurse leaders, play their part in the organization.

Front-line Nurse Leadership Restructured

It seems likely that the restructuring of nurse leadership created part of the trouble that the NUC were experiencing. Increasingly, front-line nurse leaders have become managers. Within that role, these nurses have become involved in specific new technologies of governance. We can compare this with what head nurses said about their work when interviewed by Campbell (1984) earlier. Although by 1981 all head nurses were being expected to take a course in unit management, they remained deeply involved in clinical practice. One of those head nurses mentioned her own view that head nurses should continue to do nursing care or they would lose track of therapeutic developments and their clinical skills would diminish. Another, describing her working day, said that about 50 per cent of her time was absorbed by management-type work, including committees, and the rest was spent in clinical supervision. For instance, her basic routine was to 'make rounds' and assess personally all the patients under her care every morning. However, this head nurse explained that her nursing director was encouraging head nurses to reduce their clinical activities, and she mentioned, in this regard, that 'it would be noticed' if she didn't assume leadership of committees and undertake other managerial functions. The hospital was making efforts to include their head nurses in the hospital's 'management team' and give them perks such as special education days in pleasant settings away from the hospital. Becoming a manager was already beginning to separate the head nurse from her staff – or, as we speak about it, altering her standpoint.

The move towards making head nurses into managers had taken on new dimensions by 1996 when, as part of her ethnographic data collection, Rankin followed a nursing team leader going about his job. At the beginning of his shift he methodically reviewed each patient's chart. For this front-line nurse leader, a textual review supplants the old-fashioned nursing 'rounds' in which the head nurse would personally talk to and look at every patient. As he went about his chart review, the team leader commented, 'I do this at the start of every shift so that I can stay on top of what is going on.'

By the late 1990s and into the year 2000 and beyond, much more was being changed in the work of front-line nursing leadership. Unlike staff nurses, whose job descriptions and work processes are assumed to be unchanged by restructuring, the formal descriptions of front-line nurse leaders have been undergoing revision. At the hospital where the NUC members worked, within a larger reorganization of the hospital management structure over a ten-year period, three major reviews of the front-line nursing leadership position were conducted, each with ensuing changes in title, job description, and required credentials. The head nurse disappeared, that title evolving through 'clinical coordinator,' 'nursing unit manager,' 'care coordinator,' 'team leader,' 'program manager,' and 'nurse clinician.' The changing title was part of an evolution of the nursing leadership at what we are calling the front-line of the organization – the position from which staff nurses are supervised. Judging from the numerous redefinitions of the position's title, there also seems to have been some uncertainty about the right way to structure the work of front-line nurse leaders.

Rankin's association with the NUC began during the initial move from head nurse to clinical coordinator. The job description for the new position indicated that 'under the direction of the Patient Care Manager, the Clinical Coordinator plans, organizes, coordinates, participates in and evaluates care delivery and supervises and evaluates staff on assigned unit' (Clinical Coordinator, Job Description, 1994). The new role was to include 'coordinating and ensuring the delivery of quality patient care; establishing nursing care procedures; communicating standards to staff; developing and implementing effective nursing routines; assessing workload and allocating staff accordingly;

ensuring effective discharge planning; identifying utilization issues; overseeing team conferences and unit meetings; liaising with the multidisciplinary team; carrying out quality assurance activities and projects; and advising the Patient Care Manager of ongoing deficiencies in the systems, services and resources that support patient care' (ibid).

A colloquial reading of this job description sustains the clinical interest and involvement of the clinical coordinator as it relates to effective nursing care. The job description is written in such a way that the managerial interests to which the work is now geared are not immediately apparent. It could be read as describing the pre-reform model of head nurse, where a veteran and clinically proficient nurse relies on her knowledge, skills, and personal experience to ensure that the nursing routines in her unit result in good care, that nurses' work assignments are manageable, and that members of the multidisciplinary team communicate effectively with each other. But look again. Buried in the language of this job description are traces of the text- or information-based technologies towards which this nurse leader's work is directed. As we have been demonstrating here and in previous chapters, establishing 'effective nursing routines,' 'ensuring effective discharge planning,' 'assessing workload and allocating staff,' 'identifying utilization issues,' and 'carrying out quality assurance activities and projects' – are all ineluctably linked to the specific new public management techniques of counting and comparing, classifying and categorizing, and evaluating and accounting. This job description inserts the new text-based accountability into the work of the front-line nurse leader.

A patient services manager interviewed by Rankin several years into the restructuring at the NUC hospital discussed the transitions faced by front-line nursing leadership as the position evolved into 'team leader.' The manager's comments suggest how the position was being developed to reinforce hospital efficiencies. Here she is speaking about hospital bed utilization when she says:

'We are developing the team leader role in that direction now. They [team leaders] are doing a lot better at it this year than they were last year. In fact, two of the new team leaders are actually the displaced utilization reviewers, so in that respect, they are already very much on board with utilization but now they are in a position where they are actually able to coordinate it with patients.'

By the end of the 1990s, hospital bed utilization had become an important part of nursing work. It was being integrated into routine nursing procedures. Revising the front-line nursing leadership job is part of this broadening of nurses' responsibility for improving hospital bed utilization. The patient services manager quoted above followed up her comment that the front-line nurse leaders, now called team leaders, are 'doing a lot better this year.' She continued: 'Team leaders are responsible for discharge planning so they have a pivotal role in coordinating all the things around discharge planning. Figuring out the family picture, the available services. Of course, they have staff feeding into that. But they coordinate it all – the social workers, the long-term care assessors, continuing care. They are supposed to monitor their own bed utilization.'

The team leader is responsible for coordinating discharges so that they are timely and, importantly, so that they can be tracked in utilization statistics that she and other nurse leaders will be monitoring. The excerpt above offers some insight into the nature of this work and how it is a new undertaking for nurses in front-line leadership positions. Notice also how the managerial interests in effective bed utilization motivate the whole list of activities mentioned. For instance, the team leader must 'figure out the family picture' with an interest in identifying the family member available to take on nursing responsibilities at home. Then she must understand the services that are available in the community and coordinate with the professionals involved. She is expected to organize her staff to 'feed into' the development of a comprehensive knowledge of the patent's family, financial circumstances, living situation, and so on. Team leading directed towards the execution of these responsibilities looks entirely different from the orientation of the head nurse of old. It now begins to make sense why the team leader or clinical coordinator didn't pay attention to some of the clinical issues that the NUC expected her to.

During one of her observations of a shift-change report, Rankin noticed that the team leader stopped the audiotape three times to draw nurses' attention to what she considered essential elements of their work. All three interjections were directions to her staff to ensure appropriate discharge work. For instance, she emphasized the special teaching required for patients being discharged who needed to learn to self-administer anticoagulant injections. In an aside to the researcher, the team leader said 'the new staff need to remember to teach the patients how to do it or else they have to stay an extra day, or else we have to send Home Care in.' In the past, such a reminder might have been made to coach a novice nurse on her nursing responsibilities for patients, whereas now its rationale is the thorny issue of bed utilization. If patients have not mastered the injection technique, they may require an extra – and wasteful – day in hospital. Home Care nurses might be called on, but the team leader will know that they may not be available when needed, or at all, given the rising demand for follow-up of acute patients in the community. It is the team leader's responsibility to ensure that bed-freeing activity is prioritized within the nurse's plan of care, even though it is time-consuming and takes the nurse away from other pressing acute care. The team leader's reminder about teaching patients, and maybe family members, too, how to give injections is just one of the myriad tasks that contribute to how nursing staff are being organized to 'feed into' the organizational imperative of discharge.

The contemporary front-line nurse leader has a new managerial interest in patient records. In the past the head nurse would read a patient's chart and, particularly, nurses' narrative notes, to understand the condition of a patient. Now, with recording done increasingly in flow-charts and tick-sheets, this is less and less the case. In today's hospital settings, although the team leader is increasingly oriented to textual communication, her or his interest in the patient's record is an entirely different one. This is what Rankin noted when a team leader who was reviewing patients charts at the beginning of shift explained what he was looking for: 'I do this at the start of every shift so that I can stay on top of what is going on. I need to figure out who might go.' Not only was he primarily interested in potential discharges, not clinical progress per se, but he was thinking about the nursing action that would need to be taken as the next step towards the discharge. While looking through each document, he made additional notes on his bed map and worksheet explaining, 'A big part of my job is getting the families on board early.' His talk illustrates how his clinical expertise was immediately converted into ideas about taking particularly focused action. As he quickly scanned the charts he commented on each patient, as follows: 'This patient is complex; she had a CVA [stroke] and a recent MI [heart attack]; she has liver metastasis [cancer]; she has a husband but there are no supports' ... This is a social admission – 'failure to cope.' Penny [social worker] will be ticked off, but if we need a cardiac bed that will be the first one [to go]; he really should be designated ALC ... Her son is in [small town]; that's important ... This patient lives alone in [small town]; he has a son in [big city] ... These are the difficult ones. The frail elderly fractures. She has a niece who lives in [big city] ... This elderly gentleman only has a brother – that does not bode well.'

This team leader was making judgments and decisions about his patients and their clinical conditions, but his professional expertise was focused towards *managerial* concerns. In his reading of the patients' records, no discernible clinical interest was directed to the actual nursing care required or given for the patient suffering from a stroke, a heart attack, and cancer, nor to the experiences of elderly brothers coping with an unexpected hospitalization. His focus was strictly on managing scarce bed resources as he determined 'who might go home.' It is apparent that his interest in families was related to whether they would be able to help him accomplish the discharges that he had to make. He focused on patients as units of resource utilization. His interest in clinical data was related to what tests patients were waiting for, the results of diagnostic evaluations, or the doctors' 'progress' notes. He used these clinical data to assess patients' possible trajectory – continued hospitalization, ALC designation, transfer off the unit, or a discharge home. Bed maps, patients' admission records, and bed status reports[2] are the tools that he was using to 'get on top of what is going on.'

A front-line nurse leader's work need not be exclusively focused on finding beds or organizing nursing labour. However, as this set of observations shows, these are the concerns that dominated much of this team leader's work and thinking. Any other work will be squeezed into the time left over from the work of finding beds and other managerial work. Was it this sort of organization of their team leader's time and attention that the NUC were responding to so unhappily? Their discomfort with the loss of clinical leadership becomes more and more understandable as we begin to identify what team leaders are doing in the nursing work setting.

Managing the Changing Work Relations among Nurses: Virtual Accounts

Through several chapters, we have been drawing attention to how the accounts generated in various information systems may differ from what nurses know experientially. This is true for nurses but even more so for nurse leaders. Front-line nurse leaders are positioned to straddle a 'line of fault' (Smith 1987) between the virtual reality of the management technologies and the everyday knowledge that is available, used, and trusted by nurses and doctors. Disjunctures appear between the different ways of knowing, and when they do they must be managed, if decisions about health care are to be standardized in line with health reform policy and good organizational management. Front-line nurse leaders work at the 'interchange' point (Pence 2001), where differences appear and where they are converted into organizational concepts that make them manageable. As described within official job descriptions, the work of front-line nurse leaders includes responsibilities for 'utilization,' 'quality assurance,' and the implementation of 'effective nursing care routines.' It is their responsibility to see that authorized views prevail, facilitating the imposition of objective, textually mediated, reform policy–oriented practices into the local setting. Professional judgement and care activities within the nursing unit are to be brought within the purview of authorized organizational goals – as expressed (or at least covered in) the organizational mission statement and the family of program and personnel documents that elaborate these statements as job descriptions, objectives, strategic directions, and so forth. This is a ruling function.

New concepts of leadership and methods of management borrowed from the private sector have been adopted in hospitals, such as the next example we offer where front-line nurse leaders' 'motivation' was being stimulated through generating a sense of competition. We encountered models of interdepartmental competitiveness being used in several hospitals to motivate nurses towards organizational goals more aggressively. The following instance comes from the experiences of a nurse informant who works in a hospital that contracts with an American company for its MCAP^{TM} bed utilization program. Using its virtual representation of bed availability, collective decisions are made about admissions. Our nurse informant explained how the MCAP^{TM} system of 'off index' days engaged front-line nurse leaders (here called 'clinicians') in competitive relations: 'Each day we have a 'bed meeting.' All the clinicians gather in a little room and we report which beds we have managed to clear. Then the waiting patients are doled out amongst much haggling about workload and off index' (e-mail communication, April 2000).

In the MCAP^{TM} system 'off-index' days equate to the 'lag days' or 'ALC' days in the lexicon of other hospitals' systems. Statistically, off-index days will add up to inefficient utilization of resources for which a clinician will be held responsible. Our informant is describing how her colleagues are reluctant to admit patients to their units whose age, social circumstances, and needs for care are constituted, within accountability systems, as inefficiencies. Within the colloquial lexicon of modern hospitals these sorts of patients are being described as having 'acopia'[3] or 'revolving door syndrome' as their access to care becomes increasingly contentious. Our informant explained the 'haggling' front-line nurse leaders engage in to avoid taking on these patients, saying: 'Each month all of the clinicians and the physicians wait with bated breath to see how many 'off-index' days we had. The implication being of course that the doctor is a *'bad'* doctor if he has too many off-index patient days and that the clinician on the ward is not doing the job of 'moving her patients out' appropriately if we had too many 'off-index' days' (e-mail communication, April 2000).

Nurses in front-line nursing leadership positions are held accountable to the new 'facts' generated through the technologies of counting. Through technologies such as the MCAP^{TM} system described here, the clinician's day-to-day practices of managing patients (and enforcing her staff nurses' compliance with discharge practices) can be publicly scrutinized and compared. This constructs the milieu as competitive,[4] and the clinicians involved are judged according to how they 'measure up' to the established standards – in length-of-stay data that has been objectively calculated. It has to be recognized that a strategy such as this works by encouraging these nurse leaders rather forcefully to subordinate any competing clinical values to the managerial objective of reducing length of hospital stays. (It simultaneously raises concerns about the elderly patient complaining of pain who is thought of as a potential bed blocker.)

Another interaction with a team leader during Rankin's participant observation highlighted the pressures, responsibilities, and frustrations that the nurse experienced under the scrutiny of the group she referred to as 'the bed police': 'On Thursday last week, it was so bad, we had two urgent meetings with all the team leaders, admitting and bed utilization clerks ('the bed police'). There were patients tucked into all the corners and closets of the hospital. Everybody was over census. I had been desperately looking for beds all day. I was frustrated because on my ward there was a vaginal hysterectomy who should have been sent home. We weren't doing anything for her except feeding her Tylenol #3's but her doctor had been in at 8 a.m. that morning and she (the patient) had convinced him that she wasn't yet ready to go.'

In this situation the patient and her physician, having found reasons for extending the patient's stay in the hospital, have disrupted the discharge. The clinical pathway for vaginal hysterectomy and the discharge planning have not been successfully adhered to. The front-line nurse leader reported how she was unable to negotiate the required discharge. And as a result, her competence was questioned: 'Later in the afternoon, when we had the second meeting, I was really on the line. He [the surgeon] had not been answering his pager and the ward was really going crazy. When they [the bed police] called us all back down I had to report that I had not been able to empty that bed. I knew they were not impressed, but I have to tell myself, I did everything I could.'

Occasions such as the one this nurse described placed her on the management side of the 'line of fault.' This nurse's attendance at a meeting with the 'bed police' drew her attention to the dire shortage of beds throughout the hospital. In addition, she was also caught up in the physical demands of having 'patients tucked into all corners of the hospital.' She was pulled into, and made responsible for, the added burden this creates for the staff. Through this work we see how she was strategically positioned to embrace the authorizing technologies that offered her increased sway over the recalcitrance of this physician or of other members of the professional team who delayed anticipated discharges. We see how the new technologies assisted her in reframing competent practice, even though it was a very different sort of competence from the kind Campbell's head nurse informants described in the 1980s.

The framing of the competence of front-line nurse leaders is now organized from outside the work of the ward to a greater extent than in the past. Prior to the advent of the new technologies, a head nurse's proficiency was judged through her relationships with nurses and physicians, as well as her clinical know-how. Respect was won by a head nurse's ability to use her advanced clinical expertise and organizational savvy to support the work on her ward. Also when head nurses relied on staff nurses to know what was going on with patients (rather than the textual reliance on clinical pathways, case-status designations, and chart forms of today's workplace), both levels of nurses were involved in a more reciprocal, more collegial, partnership of care. Those head nurses worked closely with and trained their staffs, knowing that their own success depended on their nurses' knowledge, skill, and willingness to work hard.

Shifting Authority: Changing Relationships

The new job descriptions and responsibilities reflect the kinds of accountability arising in information-based management technologies that now direct the front-line nurse leader's work. Today's nurse leaders are expected to be responsible for how staff nurses and other health workers use hospital resources. However, not all nurses or doctors adopt the 'efficiency' model or a cost orientation as the guide for their practice. Some, such as the gynaecologist in the previous excerpt (who allowed his patient to exceed her expected length of stay and then did not answer his pager), may hold notions about good use of time and hospital supplies and beds that differ from the managerial perspective being promulgated through the flow-sheets and clinical pathways. It becomes part of the nurse leader's job to manage not just nurses but also the intransigence of doctors, who remain entrenched in their pre-restructuring ideas. Front-line nurse leaders must win doctors' compliance with standard length of stay and achieve punctual discharges.

Managing Physicians' Resistance

Throughout the hospital reforms of the 1980s and 1990s doctors have stood in strong opposition to managerial incursions into their professional autonomy and have consistently resisted attempts to monitor and control their billing practices (Armstrong et al. 1994: 23). But the new technologies have begun to influence physicians' actions, especially regarding bed utilization and length of stay, as we shall see here. It is not easy, but the front-line nurse leaders have no option but to draw physicians into their continual search for beds. A patient services manager explained how the nurses coped with this work:

> Recently I've had to work with a couple of team leaders who are really frustrated about their role. It's about the treatment that they receive from physicians because physicians can be awkward. They want their patient to stay. These patients being sent home probably means more work for the physicians. But one of the team leaders says, 'This patient really is ready to go home; they are just waiting for that ERCP [endoscopic retrograde cholangio-pancreatography]. I suggest you send the patient home today and book the ERCP as an outpatient.' Unfortunately some of the

physicians can be difficult and it breaks down their working relationships a little bit.

Physicians have a privileged relationship within the hospital; most are not employed by the hospital and are not as susceptible to managerial authority as are employees. The nurse manager, above, spoke of 'working relationships' that the team leader had with the physicians who admitted, treated, and discharged patients from her ward. It is within those relationships that front-line nurse leaders must influence physicians' actions – and this is demanding, complicated, stressful, and highly political work. Yet, when the team leader is held accountable for her ward's bed utilization, she has to free those beds. A front-line nurse leader talked about the politics involved when she attempted to reduce doctors' use of resources by organizing a patient's discharge:

> It is us that have to be the hammers to say to the docs 'why is this patient here?' And you know, I always did that, and sometimes there would be certain physicians who were really bad about it. I could almost see them shudder when I approached because they knew I was going to ask the question. I didn't like that, because I don't want to be ... like, the nag. I want to say: 'How can we work together? What piece of information do you have that I don't? You know this person in the community. What can you tell me about why this person still needs to be here?' That is how I [have] tried to put it. But I'm not always that successful and I'm sure I come across as being the big heavy hammer, too, sometimes.

Technologies that systematically determine whether patients meet specific 'criteria' that warrant hospitalization are authoritative tools that front-line nurse leaders use to address the doctor and nurse power imbalance. Nurses support the use of these sorts of technologies, discovering that the authorizing features of numerically based data give them some sway within their thorny professional relationships with physicians. In Chapter 2 we noted that nurses employing ADT-generated information found that its use helped solve the 'relationship' problems that arose when they had to influence a doctor to discharge his patient. We reported there on one team leader who was pleased with the results she got from using comparative figures to convince an 'older' surgeon to make earlier discharges. When she was able to show him how his cases stayed in the hospital longer, on average, than those of his orthopaedic colleagues, her knowledge took on the appearance of technical expertise and was not simply a matter of a nurse contradicting or advising a doctor. While success with the doctors has the objective of freeing a bed and reducing per patient costs, there is even more at stake for front-line nurse leaders. As we discussed in the previous section, handling doctors' reluctance to discharge patients gets chalked up as nurses' competence or incompetence.

Daily, the imperative of front-line nurse leaders is to encourage the doctors and nurses with whom they are working to choose the most efficient trajectories of patient care. In large part, this is inscribed in decisions made through technologies such as workload indexing, patient classification, clinical pathways, and ALC. Added to that list are calculations and comparisons of patients' average and actual lengths of stay and bed utilization figures generated through the ADT system. That is what we mean when we say that professional nursing knowledge is being reframed through the authority of accounts that can be compared and costed. The new knowledge carries managerial weight in suggesting appropriate actions to be taken to improve efficiency and reduce per patient hospital costs. But, as we have also been showing, patient discharges are exceptional in the new actions nurses undertake. They cannot be managed directly in relation to texts; they always depend on the discretion of individual physicians and their compliance with the restructuring agenda. In addition, behind-the-scenes, is individual nurses' knowledgeable work of expediting discharges. We turn now to several instances of behind the scenes coaching and monitoring that illustrate how front-line nurse leaders also develop nurses' professional knowledge, aligning it with the restructuring agenda.

Managing Nurses' Resistance

During Rankin's observations, a complex protocol was developed to assist nurses to correctly complete a 'discharge planning' section of the hospital admission and social history form. Getting nurses to use the tool and fill out the form appropriately was a focus of nursing resistance that front-line nurse leaders had to learn to deal with. In this instance, we examine how altering nurses' interpretation of discharge planning was the means used to encourage nurses to comply. The site of resistance was located in the discharge planning documentation on the patients' admission form. At issue was a textual practice intended to expedite the work of freeing up beds. Referring to a complex protocol developed into a flow-chart, nurses (and other practitioners) were directed to make notations on the admission form that would initiate 'automatic referrals' for certain patients. Patients who met the predetermined criteria listed on the flow-chart would be referred to the appropriate discipline and/or program. For example, on admission, a patient identified as 'indigent or transient' would warrant an automatic referral to a social worker, as would a patient over the age of sixty-five who lives alone or with a frail caregiver. A patient who is 'thin, frail, or fails to thrive' would be automatically referred to 'Clinical Nutrition.' The discharge planning flow-chart protocol was intended to build time-saving efficiencies into the 'social' work necessary to move patients out of the hospital and in that way accomplish what the clinical pathway, discussed earlier, did in clinical treatment. It streamlined the processing of patients by categorizing and standardizing aspects of what they might later need.

For nurses whose main job is giving clinical nursing care, completing the admission and social history form and/or consulting the discharge planning flow-chart is not a priority. It is an add-on to their already cramped work day. Nurses who remain entrenched in their clinical practice interests must be coached to accept the importance of making room in their busy day to write up this and various other management-focused texts. It becomes a responsibility of the team leader to engage their efforts and, as we now show, a solution to filling out the discharge planning form was found. Framing the discharge planning flow-chart within a well-accepted nursing concept accomplishes something on behalf of the managerial strategy (as did a 'gerontological framing' of ALC, discussed previously). It appropriates an accepted nursing ideal for a restructuring purpose. Rankin observed one element of the necessary coaching and monitoring as a team leader reviewed patients' charts during the initial part of his shift. Glancing through the papers of a patient whose admitting diagnosis was entered as 'failure to cope,' he paused to point out the discharge section of the admission form. He nodded affirmatively, saying, 'That's good, the sheet has been done; that is one of the things I am really trying to work on with the nurses. It gets the referral process moving quickly.'

Rankin learned that the front-line nurse leaders, as a group, had also been 'working on' the problem, and she read the minutes of a meeting that had been convened around the problem of nurses not consistently using the discharge planning flow-chart. Despite the 'quick glance' design of the flow-chart, and the apparent brevity of the required charting on the discharge section of the admitting form, not many were being completed or completed properly. More reinforcement seemed necessary to ensure that nurses consistently filled in the standardized fields on the form. It is this managerial work that the team leader was referring to, above, when he commented, 'That is one of the things I am really trying to work on with the nurses.' The minutes of one meeting offer more detail about the nature of this coaching work, and here we are highlighting how the nursing concept of 'holism' is borrowed to reinforce discharge planning. As we see below, there has been a suggestion to teach nurses to understand expeditious discharges as 'holistic care.' Activating the nursing discourse in this manner is one way that team leaders 'work on' nurses' reluctance to adopt the attitude to their work that hospital restructuring calls for: 'We need education to help nurses see the significance of the social history in provision of holistic care ... Some nursing staff do not feel it [completing the discharge planning fields on the admission form] is relevant to their work with patients' (Minutes, Discharge Planning Meeting, 1995).

Terms such as 'holistic' call up a nursing framework that appeals to nurses' (and team leaders') traditional interests in patient care.[5] Holistic care 'is an example of an abstract theoretical concept that is professionally sanctioned in nursing. Holism is written about in nursing texts as 'the physical, emotional, social, economic and spiritual needs of the person' (Potter and Perry 1997: 1485). As an abstraction, holism does not describe actual activities, such as those undertaken by a nurse Rankin observed who had gone to great lengths to assist an elderly patient, even taking time to make satisfactory arrangements for the care of the patient's dog that had been left unattended because of the patient's hospitalization. Here, this nurse tried to identify whatever might reduce a patient's worries so that she could reserve her energy for her recovery. It is these sorts of nursing activities that the nursing concept of holism refers to.

Through interpreting the discharge flow-chart within the concept of holistic care, nurses are coached to attend to the patient's home context and to identify available supports as well as barriers to the patient's ability to manage at home. These tasks also seem to fit with nurses' notion of holism. But now a restructuring interest is added. A so-called holistic practice is to organize the work of completing a bureaucratic form that, in turn, initiates 'automatic referrals' for particular patients who, according to such texts, meet certain pre-established criteria. The nurse's form-filling work expedites discharges, attends to 'bed pressures,' and increases the hospital's productivity. But notice the differences. Nurses' involvement, on a patient's admission, in filling out a referral form does not necessarily recognize and treat the patient as an individual with complex characteristics and needs. Instead, it processes the patient in a bureaucratic manner. This is the ruling relation within which the nursing discourse on 'holism' is being harnessed. Nurses are being held to a new interpretation of their own standards. In this manner, the front-line nurse leaders use their nursing knowledge to rationalize and enforce nurses' compliance with the discharge planning work.

Nurses' resistance to new work requirements must be managed in new ways in restructured workplaces. The interpersonal relations between staff nurses and front-line nurse leaders are significantly altered by their involvement in the restructured approaches to hospital and nursing management; the earlier forms of collaborative work have been eroded. The reconfiguration of the work of the front-line nurse leader has been a long-term project. Since the mid-1970s, when budgeting began to be transferred to the nursing unit level, head nurses have had to learn to 'manage' their staffs. As head nurses were required to manage their staffing budgets and treat their staffs as resources to be managed, their relations were transformed. The visibility of a head nurse's success or failure, measured in terms of how she manages her staffing budget, forced head nurses to pressure their staffs. That is one way that the working relationship between a head nurse and her staff changed from a collaborative and supervisory relationship to a managerial one. Front-line nurse leaders' attention to the nursing staff is now increasingly focused on how nurses fulfil the requirements of the new efficiency mandate and its documentation. This is how the standpoint of front-line nurse leaders is organized differently from that of their head nurse predecessors and their contemporary nursing subordinates.

Within these competing expectations, tensions and problems are generated for front-line nurse leaders (and staff nurses) to resolve. Throughout Chapter 4 we have been showing how managing for efficiency has been written into front-line nurse leaders' restructured work. In the following chapter we do not leave staff nurses or front-line nurse leaders behind when our gaze turns from the ruling relations of utilization technologies to related technologies of 'quality' (such as those the NUC were adhering to when they worked on the QA forms). More needs to be said about the ruling relation being organized in the use of hospital performance reviews to which front-line nurse leaders and their staff must adhere. In Chapter 5, grounded in yet another local site of everyday activity in a contemporary hospital care, we explicate 'quality' and 'patient satisfaction' where we uncover a new emphasis on customer relations to which front-line nurse leaders (among others) must respond. We elaborate on the managerial usefulness of technologies such as these that suppress divergent views and standardize within the restructuring agenda what is to be known about hospitals.

5 Patient Satisfaction and the Management of Quality

This chapter considers quality in health care, especially how quality as a management concept differs from quality as nurses might understand good, or good enough, care. Everyone wants the provision of health care to be adequate or better. In this chapter we analyse some current efforts to improve hospital services through managerial technologies. As in the previous chapter, we focus on how things to be managed are known, by whom, and for what purposes. Here we analyse quality management, seeing it as a strategy for quality improvement guided by textual practices of tracking, classification, and evaluation that constitute 'quality of care,' virtually. Maintaining our interest in what actually happens to patients, our research makes use of ethnographic data that introduce and question the quality of care a patient experiences within a contemporary health care workplace.

Janet Rankin was on the scene when her aunt had to be hospitalized. She was called on to act, first as a professional nurse, and then as family caregiver to a hospitalized patient. Subsequently, Janet and her aunt responded to a patient and family survey addressing the quality of the hospital care. We work here from the data that all these experiences provide, and our argument has several strands. At the outset, we look into what Janet recognized as troubling gaps in the care given to her aunt, and we 'listen in' as Janet and her aunt attempt to answer questions about their experiences in the posthospitalization survey. Then we show how patient and family surveys such as this one become part of 'patient satisfaction,' information that advances a hospital's quality improvement strategy. From our ethnographic data we see just how difficult it is to adequately represent the actualities of health care in text, but nevertheless survey findings become a definitive account.

Procedures such as this generate the abstractions – including the rankings, statistical indicators, and outcomes – that under the new public management would guide organizational action towards quality care. In previous chapters we have argued that even though the restructuring of health care may improve its efficiency, it also undermines nurses' own capacity to engage with their patients as knowledgeable professionals. We have been critical of that. Here we begin, similarly, to dissect quality improvement in health care – the application of particular technologies for managing a work process. We show that quality manifested as a ruling concept within the new public management of health care is an entirely different matter from adequate nursing care. But our critique goes much further than that. We cast doubt on the adequacy of care that can result when trust in its quality is placed in virtual accounts that have been constituted for a specific management purpose. Organized to accomplish a ruling agenda, the form of knowing 'quality' being generated suppresses the voice and standpoint of those 'on the ground' – nurses, patients, and families who are the subjects of health care. We argue that this should be a matter of considerable concern for the practice of health care.

An Urgent Hospitalization: An Account from a Patient and Family Perspective

Janet, a nursing instructor from Vancouver Island, has flown to the interior of British Columbia to spend the Easter weekend with her seventy-year-old Aunt Hannah. The much anticipated family weekend is disrupted by Hannah's accidental fall down a flight of stairs. Janet discovers her aunt unconscious in the basement, with a pool of blood around her head. Instead of the planned family brunch, Janet finds herself calling 911 and assisting the ambulance attendants to apply a rigid neck collar before transferring her aunt onto a stretcher and then helping to carry her up the steep stairway. At the small local hospital Hannah is rapidly assessed as having potentially serious neck and head injuries, and she needs to be moved to a larger regional hospital, which is a two-hour drive away. Janet stands in (on this holiday weekend with no local staff available) for the required Registered Nurse to accompany a patient on such a transfer. Janet thus finds herself pulled into the unfolding drama of an interface with the Canadian health care system from a vantage point different from that of either a nursing instructor or researcher.

At the regional hospital the emergency computer-assisted tomography (CAT) scan rules out spinal cord injury, but reveals a serious head injury – a subdural hematoma. Hannah requires transfer to a large tertiary care centre with a neurosurgery program. Within hours, Hannah is moved by air ambulance to the coast. In the meantime, the social worker in the emergency room of the regional hospital assists Janet to alter her own travel arrangements so that she can be with her aunt. Somewhat magically, it seems to Janet, her original ticket has been exchanged, and she is offered a seat on the next available flight.

This is Janet's account of the events leading up to Hannah's ten-day hospitalization. It reflects impressively prompt access to medical intervention. And at the tertiary care centre Hannah received ready access to a magnetic resonance imaging (MRI) machine and consultation from a neurosurgeon who determined that she would not require surgical intervention. During her aunt's hospitalization, Janet spent many hours at her bedside and, from the beginning, she was more active in Hannah's care than a non-professional family member would have been. Janet was able to observe the nursing care Hannah was given, some instances of which, in her professional opinion, were implicated in the complications that marred her recovery period. In the end, Hannah recovered full consciousness, was discharged home, and over the next few months she successfully rehabilitated, adapting quite well to the mild long-term deficits caused by her head injury. Despite this 'happy ending,' the occasions in which Janet saw serious gaps in Hannah's care are deserving of further study.

Troubling Gaps in Patient Care

Janet's observations included the following glimpses of Hannah's condition and her progress. During the early days of her hospitalization Hannah experienced low serum sodium (a not uncommon response to a severe head injury). As a result she was placed on a fluid restriction of 800 mL a day. During this time Janet noticed that minimal nursing attention was given to measuring Hannah's fluid intake or her urine output. There was an 'Intake and Output' record posted by the door to her room, but the staff picking up her meal trays or cleaning the cups away from her bedside were not professional nurses, and therefore information about her intake of fluids was routinely missed. Likewise, when Hannah went to the bathroom, she was seldom assisted by the same nurse twice, and no one was monitoring the volume of her output of urine. Janet had concerns about what this lack of nursing attention to Hannah's fluid balance meant for her health, in view of the fact that while her fluid intake was being severely restricted, she was also experiencing a virulent bladder infection. On one occasion, during an afternoon visit, Hannah mentioned to Janet that she had not urinated since early the previous morning (approximately 32 hours ago). The 'Intake and Output' record had nothing written on it for the previous 24 hours. Janet assisted her aunt to the bathroom where, with appropriate 'nursing intervention' (such as running water, reflex stimulation, privacy) she passed 900 mL of very foul-smelling, concentrated, urine. Hannah's overly full bladder may have contributed to her persistent fever, her overnight restlessness (and subsequent physical restraint), and her mild confusion.

Janet believed that inattention to Hannah's intake and output, while she also had a severe bladder infection and was on fluid restriction for another condition, signified a serious omission in her daily nursing care. Besides that, Janet considered that lack of attention to Hannah's fluid consumption and her urine output may also have contributed to yet another problem, a flare-up of Hannah's heart condition. On a second occasion of Hannah's overly full bladder being overlooked, she required urgent transfer to a cardiac intensive care unit. Hannah had a pre-existing cardiac condition known as paroxysmal superventricular tachycardia. Prior to her accident, her cardiac condition had been stabilized with medication. On this occasion, the noxious stimulus of Hannah's overly full bladder most likely contributed to the triggering events that caused her normally stable condition to become unstable. An intensive care nurse detected the full bladder shortly after Hannah had been transferred into the cardiac care unit. This nurse inserted a urinary catheter and drained 1,000 cc of urine from Hannah's bladder. Hannah's serious cardiac arrhythmia did not respond to three attempts of cardioversion with electrically charged chest paddles. Eventually she was placed on intravenous Amiodarone, an anti-arrhythmic drug. In the meantime she suffered abrasions on her chest as a result of the cardioversion attempts. Janet recognized that this potentially avoidable situation seriously jeopardized Hannah and contributed to her overall discomfort and suffering.

Janet's observations and interactions with the nursing staff also gave her cause for concern. Janet was with Hannah on the neuroscience ward early in the morning when Hannah's arrhythmia developed.[1] That morning, the nurse caring for Hannah was a recent graduate, a casual employee. Janet noticed that he seemed overburdened with the needs of the patients in Hannah's four-bed ward. When Janet called him to report her aunt's racing pulse and complaints of feeling 'woozy' he was completing his night shift. He did not assess Hannah. Instead he informed Janet that he had just taken Hannah's vital signs and that she was fine. Unconvinced, Janet quickly located a stethoscope and, upon finding Hannah's blood pressure had dropped significantly, was able to convince the nurse to call a doctor. Throughout Janet's experiences she was aware that nurses seemed to be irritated or possibly intimidated by her vigilance. This was a disconcerting experience for her, as her own beliefs and training directed her to be a 'good family member' while visiting her aunt. She worked hard to stay out of the nurses' way while contributing to her aunt's care as much as possible. Yet, as in this case, Janet drew to their attention to any issues that she thought they would want to know.

Janet was not satisfied with her interaction with Hannah's assigned nurses, and she had no better success trying to consult with the unit's nurse leader. The following story from her notes illustrates this. Janet had observed that the order for severe (800 cc per day) fluid restriction issued for Hannah had not been reviewed for several days. Worried about Hannah's complaints of significant thirst, Janet approached the nursing desk and asked to review the laboratory results of a daily sodium test. She was referred to the manager of the clinical practice unit who was called from her office, which was located some distance from the unit, to speak to Janet. The manager tried to be helpful, but she explained that family access to this sort of information is restricted until someone (presumably a physician) is available to explain and interpret it authoritatively. Here, Janet recognized that her interest in Hannah's complaints of thirst became, for the manager, an administrative concern about a family's appropriate access to hospital documents. Thus, on this occasion, despite the fact that the manager was a nurse, she did not take up clinically Janet's questions about the care of a patient on her unit, and she did not respond satisfactorily to Janet's concerns.

The Patient and Family Surveys

Three months following Hannah's discharge from hospital she was mailed a package of survey materials. It included an introductory letter, an 18-page booklet, called *Through the Patient's Eyes: Patient Survey*, and a shorter survey questionnaire for a family member involved with the hospitalization. The letter explained that Hannah's name had been drawn from a random sample of patients admitted to the hospital. The surveys invited Hannah and her family to give feedback about their hospital experience. The Patient Satisfaction Survey asked 127 questions under ten categories such as: Communication and Relationships, Your Daily Care, Preparation for Discharge, and so forth. Generally the questions offered forced choices 'strongly agree,' 'agree,' 'uncertain,' 'disagree,' and 'strongly disagree,' or 'excellent,' 'very good,' 'good,' 'fair,' and 'poor' (see Figure 5.1). The surveys were to be filled out by both the patient and the most involved family member. So, when Hannah requested Janet's assistance with the Patient Survey, Janet once again travelled to her aunt's home to help.

Hannah and Janet both willingly participated in the surveys. They thought it was important to give feedback about 'how [The Hospital][2] staff are doing' as the surveys' introduction asked. They both had things to say, appreciative and critical, that they thought would help in the hospital's undertaking to 'improve the delivery of health care to you and your family' (quoted from the surveys' introduction). They completed the surveys together, consulting with one another, remembering the hospital experience, and trying to give an accurate account. But doing so was not a straightforward endeavour. Hannah couldn't answer questions about her admission to the hospital because she was not fully conscious when she was admitted. Even some of her memories of later events were blurry. Janet, too, could not answer many of the questions on the surveys and others, not relevant to their particular experience, were of little interest to her. For instance, it was not relevant to Janet whether she and her aunt had received information related to the hospital daily routine or whether the admitting process was 'poor' or 'excellent.' Their answers to these questions were perfunctory and perhaps therefore not very accurate or revealing. Janet's needs in relation to Hannah's hospital admission had revolved around making her own travel arrangements and, upon arrival, trying anxiously to find Hannah in the large metropolitan hospital. Janet recalled becoming lost when she got off an elevator in a corridor flanked by two doors, each marked 'authorized personnel only.' She could not find a place in the surveys to mention the rising panic she felt as after her already long day of anxiety, travel, and little sleep, she had wandered around the hospital looking for her aunt's room.

While the Patient Survey's 127 questions did appear to be asking about experiences of which Janet and Hannah had some knowledge, the prescribed choice of responses restricted severely what could be

Figure 5.1: Sample Page of Patient Survey

Through the Patient's Eyes

18.   When you had questions to ask a doctor, did you get answers you understood?
1.   Always
2.   Usually
3.   Sometimes
4.   Never
9.   Didn't Have Any Questions

19.   In terms of confidence and trust, please rate your relationship with the nurse(s) on your unit.
1.   Excellent
2.   Very Good
3.   Good
4.   Fair
5.   Poor

20.   Were the nurses available when you needed them?
1.   Always
2.   Usually
3.   Sometimes
4.   Never
5.   Don't Know

21.   When you had questions to ask the nurses, did you get answers you understood?
1.   Always
2.   Usually
3.   Sometimes
4.   Never
9.   Didn't Have Any Questions

22.   Were you satisfied with the way information about your condition was given to you?
1. Yes   2. No
If No, why were you not satisfied?

_____

_____

23.   How much information was your family given about your hospital care?
1.   Enough Information
2.   Too Much Information
3.   Too Little Information
9.   No Family

said. Under the heading 'Communication and Relationships' both Hannah and Janet wanted to mention how information related to Hannah's significant sensitivity to the drug nitroglycerine had not been passed on among the doctors and nurses caring for her. They wanted the hospital to know that information about Hannah's pre-existing medical conditions had somehow been lost. (Twice, she had been given nitroglycerine for complaints of chest pain, both times occasioning urgent medical intervention to support the sudden drop in her blood pressure.) Both Janet and Hannah would also have described the time when a cardiologist asked Janet to leave the room while he was examining Hannah, during which time he had mistakenly asked her about a heart surgery that she had never had. In view of Hannah's head injury and related speech difficulties this was a disconcerting and troubling experience with potential for serious error. None of these critically important details about what actually happened, things Hannah and Janet wanted to volunteer about their communication and relationships, had a place in the Patient Satisfaction Survey tool. For instance it was impossible to accurately answer the question: 'In terms of confidence and trust, please rate your relationship with the nurses(s) on your unit?' The relationships Hannah had within the various units and with the various nurses depended very much upon the acuteness of her condition and the experience and approach of the particular nurse she was encountering. Despite occasions when she had a great deal of confidence in the nurses, and times when she felt the nurses were very available to her when she needed them, Hannah responded that her confidence and trust were 'fair' and that nurses were available to her 'sometimes,' in order to account for the times when she felt the nurses had not responded to her needs.

Hannah completed the section relating to 'Daily Care' in a manner that indicated that she was 'completely satisfied.' This was her opinion. It was in this section of The Survey that Janet's responses, based on her professional education and experience, disputed her aunt's views. Even so, the responses Janet and her aunt made as they completed the patient and family satisfaction surveys did not reflect the actualities of their hospital experiences. Janet blamed this on the way that the formatting of the surveys made it impossible for them to express their concerns about what had actually happened. But this reading of the survey and its purposes was the colloquial one that patients and family members, given instructions in the accompanying material, would know how to make. We turn now to our analytic reading.

Reconstituting Knowledge about Patient Care for Accountability

Hannah and Janet were frustrated in their desire to pass on what they wanted The Hospital staff to know, and through the surveys, to help them reflect on 'how [they] are doing.' Their frustration suggests that the surveys worked differently from what they had expected – that they would be able to describe how they had *experienced* the hospitalization. If not an account of patients' and families' experiences, then what were the surveys for? Answering that question is what we turn to now. This part of our inquiry begins with Hannah and Janet completing the surveys. They entered into what Smith calls a text-reader conversation in which, unlike in spoken conversations, one side of the conversation is fixed and unresponsive to the other's replies, being 'obstinately unmoveable,' as Smith (2001: 175) notes. We have already seen how the text-reader conversation coordinated Hannah's and Janet's remembered experiences in the form-filling. For instance, The Survey's methodology *standardized* Hannah's and Janet's responses. Hannah, unasked, had written the actual name of a doctor in whom she had a great deal of confidence, and Janet had pencilled in the comment 'when requested' beside a question about the information she and Hannah received. They were trying to be specific and accurate. Despite this remedial work on it, the text fixed what they could say. Its social science methodology had already determined how concepts were operationalized and what kind of responses would be countable. Pencilled-in alterations or expansions of categories would be methodologically excluded. Such detail is not organizationally useful. Lacking standardization, it cannot be processed. The required reading of the text pulls the respondents into providing, in the precise form of reply requested, their instances of and comments on the questions the text poses. This feature of survey methodology is normally unremarkable, yet it contributes to the commensurability that is an essential element of the new public management.

The Survey's fixing of one side of the account could be said to be 'active' in specific organizational relations. Our analysis emphasizes the knowledge-based processes, usually not visible, that organizational texts such as the Patient Satisfaction Survey activate. In conducting this part of our inquiry, we assume that The Survey 'does not stand alone but is intertextually connected with a textually organized complex that can be explored ethnographically' (Smith 2001: 192). We explicate how the standardized account (as part of an organizational and intertextual complex) hooks that local setting (including Hannah's hospitalization and The Survey) into other settings and other conversations. We need to discover what is being accomplished when Hannah and Janet are hooked into the broader organizational systems at work. Smith's argument on text-reader conversations as elements of ruling practices is instructive here. 'By treating [the text-reader/respondent conversation] reflexively and embedding it in the actual social relations to which it is articulated, its (ruling) schemata can be relocated as features of social relations' (Smith 1990a: 153). Smith says of the texts she analyses that they 'feed into the construction of an objectified "reality" that is independent of and displaces particular perspectives' (2001: 176). What is the importance to nursing of displacing *its* perspective? The answer to this question will emerge as our inquiry moves from a focus on The Survey as a textual object to an explication of the relations in which The Survey arose and was used.

The Intertextual Complex for Organizing and Assuring 'Patient-centred Quality of Care'

We begin this part of our inquiry with the documents that Rankin received in response to her request to The Hospital for copies of internal documents generated by The 1998 Survey, the one that she and her aunt had filled out. Moving inward from these documents, we identify the components of an administrative intertextual complex. In the rest of the chapter, we explore how hospital activities are represented in various texts that are brought together within an accounting logic – offering managerial staff new methods of assuring quality, at least 'virtually.' This gives only a taste of the complexity that is the textual basis for contemporary hospital management and regional governance.

The Hospital gave Rankin access to a short (two-page) report entitled *In Pursuit of Quality 1998: Brief Summary* and to an excerpt (pages 16 through 20) of the full 1998 report – *In Pursuit of Quality 1998* – that contained the statistical breakdown of patients' responses to thirteen of the 127 Survey questions. A copy of an earlier patient survey, *In Pursuit of Quality: An Assessment of the Quality of Care and Quality of Worklife at [The Hospital]* (1995), that had circulated widely offered some additional insight. These documents show the recursive development of The Survey – that is, how The Survey was 'nested' in a broad set of institutional processes and documentary practices (see G. Smith 1995).[3] The repetition of the word 'quality' in all the titles emphasized the centrality of that concept. Another central concept at work was 'patient-centred care.' The 1995 summary report referred to an earlier publication entitled *Through the Patient's Eyes: Understanding and Promoting Patient-Centred Care* (Gerteis et al. 1993). The Gerteis book and its own references establish the relationship of the Survey to 'patient-centred care' and of both 'quality' and 'patient-centred care' to increasingly important ideas about 'patient satisfaction' and patients as customers. Here we ask, What are these concepts, in what social relations do they exist, and how do they work? The opening statement (reproduced here) of The Hospital's Survey repeats a sentence from the introductory letter about the hospital 'changing.' As our analysis unfolds, more features of the 'change' can be recognized within the intertextual complex. We follow where The Survey materials lead us, tracing the social relations of which they are part.

We're Changing to Make Your Stay Better

Patient centred care is at the very core of [The Hospital's] vision for the future. It is a way of organizing, designing and delivering improved programs and services to you and your family.

Your Patient Centred Care Team represents your care providers, from the cleaning staff to the doctors. The team looks at the way we are meeting your needs and concerns, such as physical comfort, emotional support, family involvement and availability of information. The team is working to improve the delivery of health care to you and your family.

This opening statement draws patients and families into The Hospital's project of quality improvement. Reading this, both Hannah and Janet wanted to contribute. We think back to Janet's complaint that their comments and responses were dominated by the form of the questions and by the 'multiple choice' categories provided for their answers. The Survey built for The Hospital *an authorized knowledge* of 'patient satisfaction' – in a form that could be worked with, processed, and compared. It worked up what patients and family members had to say, leaving behind individual concerns, such as those Hannah and Janet thought were important. When properly categorized and coded,

Hannah's and Janet's experiences joined all the other information being generated in commensurable form to 'improve the delivery of hospital care,' as The Survey said. Satisfaction rankings are crucial to the construction of quality as a commensurable object whose usefulness includes transcending actual people and their everyday particular experiences. The Survey's capacity was to generate the data for those rankings. According to Smith (2001), it is the constancy of the text that makes such an account organizationally useful; among other things, constancy overcomes the difficulty of having to address the many and shifting perspectives on quality within any organization. It is this knowledge of quality that was reported in The Hospital's summary document.

In the administration of health care, conventions for accreditation and quality management programs are realized in the intertextual complex for managing quality of care. In The Hospital, The Survey appears to be part of a process whereby specified requirements of an accredited health care facility are being put in place.[4] Procedures for matching systematic textual accounts to standards have become the internationally recognized basis for accrediting hospitals (CCHSA website 2004; Smith et al. 1999). A complex of textual representations will bring satisfaction rankings (and 'customers' priorities') together with standards of quality for other institutional purposes, too. According to public policy analyst Yamamoto, such techniques for 'improving the quality of services, setting standards for quality, and *responding to customers' priorities'* (2003: 6, emphasis added) are being drawn together and develop new emphases within the new public management.

Janet and Hannah would not have been expected to understand that the text of The Survey was establishing an interpretive frame for their experiences that would translate their comments into the 'priorities of the customer.' But in textual form, a number of new emphases are given to what they experienced. People's responses in The Survey become representations of 'what actually happens' or 'what is' – worked up into an objective information form. Measurement is the accepted way of comparing 'what actually happens' to standards, in this case, to standards of quality. Standards establish 'what the organization does to ensure that its products and services satisfy the customer's quality requirements and comply with any regulations applicable to those products or services' (ISO website 2004). 'What the organization does' in this case points to a generic set of quality management practices that include, in Hannah's health care setting, not just 'patient satisfaction' surveys, but 'patient-centred care' and other procedures that are to make use of an accounting logic. Our analysis shows that patient satisfaction becomes one measurable element of the 'quality' product or final outcome of care given in The Hospital – within the intertextual complex that stands in for what actually happens, making it manageable. Below, we examine the quality management discourse to see how patient satisfaction contributes to it. In the process we discover how ruling relations enter into nurses' work through their involvement in The Hospital's use of this related set of management practices.

Quality Management

Quality management is an approach to regulating health care outcomes that was taken up in the United States[5] in the late 1980s, its practices adapted from manufacturing, for which they had originally been designed. Transplanted into the health care sector in the United States, quality management came to the rescue of health care agencies faced with the failure of earlier methods of assuring quality of care (Rocchiccioli and Tilbury 1998: 242). Quality management was made famous by its association with Japan's postwar industrial recovery and became a movement carrying great expectations. Its contemporary place within the health care discourse reflects a similar enthusiasm. Quality management's many versions share a main feature of industrial quality control: the 'recognition, analysis and elimination of variation' in health care work processes (Laffel and Blumenthal 1993: 40). According to Rocchiccioli and Tilbury, quality management was also the chosen method of handling the new pressures of 'rising health care costs, concerns of third party payers, burgeoning technological breakthroughs in surgical techniques that shortened hospital length of stays, growth in competition and consumer demands' (1998: 242). It addresses the elusive concept of health care quality through managerial intervention, focusing on performance measured through procedural and statistical methods.[6]

One quality management expert Brian Joiner[7] claims, on behalf of these methods, that 'performance is largely determined by the system within which employees work: its policies, processes, procedures, training, equipment, instructions, materials' (1994: 33), pointing out that these are things that *only management can change.* Joiner insists that although 'individual skill, ability, and motivation are important,' they 'play a much smaller role than previously assumed' in the achievement of quality (ibid.). In Canada, the move towards performance evaluation in health care ratifies this stance. (We will argue that in this process, nurses' expertise is transformed and thus loses its import as knowledge of actual patients.)

The systematic organization of work is one important feature of quality management and its customer focus is another. Together, they identify how an organization can be successful. 'A true customer focus is being able to identify and eliminate work in our organizations that has little meaning or value to customers,' allowing the creation of systems to 'translate that knowledge about customers into strategic direction and daily action' (Joiner 1994: 62). This account of customer focus goes some way to explaining the centrality of 'patient-centred care' to the program of quality management in The Hospital. The Hospital's vision, according to the 1995 internal document, *In Pursuit of Quality: An Assessment of the Quality of Care and Quality of Worklife at [The Hospital]*, was 'to create a humane, *patient-centred*, academic health sciences centre where physicians, staff and volunteers are committed to fostering an environment that enhances the needs of our patients. One way to create such an environment is through *patient centred care'* (Preamble, emphasis added). Said to be a 'way of organizing and delivering improved programs' (The Survey, 1), patient-centred care emphasizes that the organization of what is to be done revolves around the patient as customer. As we have already indicated and will elaborate further, 'revolves around' means something quite specific – and includes accountability in cost terms.

The notion of customer (and the costing related to customers' interests) that quality management introduces into health care necessitates that the work be sequenced in a way that transforms inputs into specified final products or measurable outputs (Al-Assef and Schmele 1993). Systems, such as clinical pathways, are developed to guide and constrain practitioners' actions towards predetermined outcomes that are designed to be 'efficient,' and measurably so. Under the customer orientation, this systematic organization of action is viewed as allowing for the optimum service *for the patient*.[8] Waste can be detected in variances from clinical pathways, for instance, or in reference to any other procedure with predefined units of standard activity. The strategy of eliminating variances has broad application. Patient-centred care is said to create a common ground for everybody involved in health care. In a text reference in the introduction to The Hospital's

Survey material, Gerteis et al., discuss patient-centred care as a framework to 'provide common ground for patients worried about health and well-being, managers worried about competition and efficiency, clinicians worried about quality of care, and payers worried about cost-effectiveness to talk and work together' (1993: xiii).

This notion of a 'common ground' may be the colloquial way of saying 'commensurable' that, as we have argued, is the goal of standardization. We have already shown commensurability to be the basis in the new public management for the application of accounting logic. When patient care is scrutinized for its efficiency, the judgement takes place in a textual complex, through calculating costs. It may identify a requirement for rearrangements of space, personnel, and equipment, as well as redesign of work processes. Our reading and analysis of the intertextual complex and its related practices reveals that patient-centred care is not just an attitude of 'putting the patient first' that practitioners should adopt. It is a specific way of designing the work setting and the work itself and for conceptualizing its outcomes to make inputs and outputs available for statistical comparison. In the intertextual complex, quality and efficiency are blended.

The nursing profession has been largely uncritical of this approach. An example that comes to hand is a discussion paper on patient-centred care, or as it is sometimes called, patient-focused care, published by the Registered Nurses Association of British Columbia (1996a). Notice, in the excerpts below, the language and the aims of quality management. For instance, RNABC publications say that patient-centred care is a 'centralized' approach to care 'organized to meet the needs of the client and provided at the convenience of the client'; it is part of an 'interdisciplinary patient care delivery system.' It attempts to bring together in one unit 'a greater variety of services and personnel' (RNABC 1996a: 3). Specifically, patient-centred care is said to be based on the premise that 'multiskilling can occur among professional disciplines or between professionals and assistive personnel. Delivery of patient care within a service unit is coordinated by self-directed work teams comprising professional and assistive multiskilled health care workers' (RNABC 1996a: 5). According to the RNABC, the reported benefits of an interdisciplinary patient-care delivery system include 'improved coordination of client care, greater accountability for the effectiveness and quality of patient care, improved strategic planning [and] improved cost control' (RNABC 1996b: 3).

Whether called a centralized approach or a common ground,

patient-centred care follows the customer-oriented work organization of quality management. Whether redesigning the actual space or restructuring jobs and supervision, the goal is to reduce wasted time and effort. Protocols and procedures establish the right way to process patients and conduct their care to accomplish the reduction of variance from the approved standard. Of course, all these efforts depend entirely upon the availability of properly constituted information – describing the patient, the work, the outcome, and so forth in commensurable terms. This is where our analysis of different forms of knowing health care becomes relevant. We will have more to say presently about what it means for nurses and patients that efficiency and quality are blended in so-called objective information.

Our ethnographic data challenge the taken-for-granted goodness of care organized in this manner. For one thing, it may be difficult to discern to what extent the whole objective accounting effort actually improves a patient's treatment and recovery. Even so, there are important rhetorical uses of the new knowledge – about patient satisfaction, for instance. Because of the high public profile of health care, the evidence offered by patient satisfaction surveys finds its way into political debates. In one such instance, the leader of B.C. New Democratic opposition party accused the governing Liberals of 'inflating' health satisfaction numbers from a survey of hospital emergency departments. Zeroing in on 'mediocre marks from patients on every category' that 'magically turn into overwhelming approval of health care,' NDP leader Carol James called it a 'fantasy concocted by [the governing party]' (NDP newswire, October 2004). Although having rhetorical and partisan uses, it would be a mistake to think of the virtual realities that support the new public management as fantasies. As Smith says, 'textual realities are not fictions or falsehoods; they are normal, integral, and indeed essential features of the relations and apparatuses of ruling – state administrative apparatuses, management, professional organizations ... and so forth,' and she adds, 'these methodologies are enforced' (1990a: 83). This is why we shift our analytic gaze now towards patient satisfaction as ruling practice.

'Patient Satisfaction': Ideological Practices of Ruling

Patient satisfaction is to health care what customer focus is to a commercial firm. It is a concept from a discourse on management and, as such, reflects the shift taking place in how health care is to be properly managed. Knowing certain facts about patients' experiences (how they are constituted as levels of satisfaction) makes possible the best use of resources and other responses to influence 'quality,' outcomes, as discussed already. Like a customer focus, patient satisfaction is conceptualized as 'what patients' want,' and that knowledge is produced using social science methods. When available in the proper information form, what patients' want can be realized, for instance, through use of the organizational strategies that together can be called patient-centred care.

As a concept for ruling health care organizations and activities, patient satisfaction is *constructed* from the actualities of people's lives as patients. Or rather, the actualities of living people become a resource to be made over into the image of the concept 'patient satisfaction.' This highly developed and perfectly ordinary intellectual work Dorothy Smith calls 'ideological practice' and she associates it with the text-based ruling activities of postindustrial society (1990a: 43–5). Patient satisfaction stands in as 'what patients want.' It provides knowledge in the objectified form that is part of how success is conceptualized – as quality – and realized within the organization. Subjectivities of actual people are eliminated. Although the concept is substituted for the actuality, a 'methodical history' (Smith 1990a: 73) 'warrants the relation between the account and an actuality.'

We paraphrase Smith (1990a: 44) in the following sketch of how social science methodology and managerial discourse stand behind 'patient satisfaction,' warranting its achievement of the proper relationship between the account and the original it claims to represent. (1) Individuals are asked questions in a survey. (2) Their answers are detached from the original practical determination of the questionnaire *and* from the part that the researcher played in making them; the answers become data, while the questions do not, and the data (the responses) are coded. (3) Analytic procedures lead to statistical manipulation to determine central tendencies. (4) The original individuals are now changed into the researcher's aggregate 'patient' to whom is attributed some ranking of 'satisfaction.' Satisfaction has thus been separated from the people who were the actual patients, who knew and responded about actual situations of care. Smith (1990a), quoting Marx (1976: 107), wants us to see as *ideology* this separation of thought from the actualities of society and history, a separation that 'makes language into an independent realm' (1990a: 51). We will take up this interest in language in Chapter 6. Here we focus on the circularity being constructed, once the grounding of the concept in an actuality is dispensed with. Patient satisfaction is now grounded in the managerial discourse and carries the imprint of the theory and concepts that the researcher began with. But note that it might have drawn on another (almost any other)[9] discourse – it has 'independence' from actualities.

Of course, the particular conceptual framing of satisfaction (within the discourse of quality and patient-centred care that we have been describing) is the useful one in the managed setting. It makes possible, for ruling purposes, a 'sorting' and 'selecting' from the respondent's actuality in a hospital. The work of managing patient satisfaction is built on what has come before – the development of categories and questions and prior decisions about appropriate statistical appli-cations. The work also projects forward into future decisions and activities. We will take up the 'forward' ruling purposes of patient sat-isfaction shortly. First, we look backward at how the conceptual work-up distorts what respondents know and want to say. We can see in the methodical history of The Hospital's Patient and Family Satisfaction Surveys the ordinary intellectual work process that we refer to now as 'ideological practice' (following Smith 1990a). The Survey's categories and associated questions are adapted from the *Canadian Patient-Centred Hospital Care Study Questionnaire* and are a reconstituted (and recur-sive) form of 'seven primary dimensions' that Gerteis et al. maintain 'capture what is important to patients' (1993: 5). The discourse demon-strates how the dimensions of the Canadian questionnaire were them-selves developed in the United States using a survey and sampling technology that included a brief questionnaire administered through a telephone survey in conjunction with focus groups with physicians and non-physician hospital staff, as well as a review of the 'pertinent literature to help flesh out the context of the patient's observations' (1993: 5). The researcher uses The Survey and focus group data to develop a framework of concepts said to represent what patients want: '(1) respect for patients' values, preferences, and expressed needs; (2) coordination and integration of care; (3) information, communication and education; (4) physical comfort; (5) emotional support and allevia-tion of anxiety; (6) involvement of family and friends; and (7) transi-tion and continuity' (1993: 5–11). These dimensions both inform managerial strategies that will fulfil them (patient-centred care) and circle round to generate the questions and the patient responses about the way the hospital works (patient satisfaction/quality). That is where Hannah and Janet encountered them. The Patient and Family

Surveys' categories constructed equivalence between the concepts of the theory of 'what patients want' (already discursively available) and themselves – actual patients and their experiences, now being generated quantitatively. An actuality (that a patient or family respondent recollects when she responds to a question in The Survey) will 'automatically' become an expression of the concept. Aggregated and calculated, this process eventually arrives at a ranking of 'patient satisfaction.'

Yet the journey from a patient's experience to virtual and ideal representation to ruling practice is fraught with difficulty, at least for the respondents. Our ethnographic data show that Hannah and Janet struggled to express what they wanted to say. The Survey seems to have a mind of its own. Although they may have wanted to express themselves differently from the way the questions were asked, the structure of The Survey maintained control over their responses. The Survey's methods of inscription were not treated as features of the textual reality – those questions were 'fixed,' and they shaped what could be said; nevertheless, we have noted that the questions were not treated as data – only the answers were. Even though Hannah could express clearly her experiences of difficulty in interacting with the nurses, her categorized comment, no matter what she wished to say, became an element of the predetermined concept. Any choice of response to a question framed within 'Relationships with Nurses' would be understood within that framework, *where it would be read for whatever it already represented.* It may be treated as evidence about the nature of the personal relationship established between nurses and their patients. (Indeed, we can imagine that data like this might suggest to an enthusiastic nurse manager that she institute a campaign for nurses to smile more.)[10] Janet or Hannah ticking 'fair' or poor' would affect how the nurse-patient relationship was rated. But there would be no connection made between the frustration and anxiety that Hannah and Janet experienced when they could not get a nurse to listen to concerns about Hannah's racing heart, nor what that might have meant for the success of the ward's organization. The connections were predetermined within the customer framework already established.

But remember what was going on that morning as Hannah and Janet tried to get the weary night nurse to attend to Hannah's feelings of wooziness. This is what Hannah might have been recollecting as she attempted to answer the question about relationships with nurses. Her response 'Fair' would be coded and aggregated, nevertheless, and establish whether patients are getting what they want. There is no going back to the actuality to see how Janet's talking (or not) with a nurse would have been instrumental in Hannah's care. No insight is to be gained about how the self-managed team failed this patient. Janet's contribution to the hospital's knowledge could only be as The Survey preconceptualized and reconstituted it. Of course, The Survey design guarantees the validity and reliability of the instrument[11] – but at the same time, what we have in the end is a textual representation that fails to express Hannah's and Janet's experiences. The achievement is an account of what actually happened or what actually *is* that, according to Smith (1990a), has a circular and ideological structure. And it will carry real weight.

We signalled earlier that patient satisfaction has a part to play in ruling. It represents a very important change in how hospitals think about quality, how to capture an adequate account of quality, and how to improve it. All this shifts into the sphere of managerial responsibility. Implemented in programs of patient-centred care, knowing 'what patients want' appear to offer much more control over many aspects of patient care than is ordinarily possible (*CNA* 1993). When an ideal representation replaces all those various concerns that individual patients might voice, covering 'what patients want' can be accomplished much more efficiently through programmed managerial efforts. Of course, as noted earlier, the concept of having care revolve around the patient includes making cost savings, too. And, as reported by *CNA* (1993), one hospital patient-centred program not just satisfies patients, but 'is serving more patients with an enhanced quality of care, with no budget increases' (ibid.: Fact Sheet Two).

Enhancing the capacity to rule is a different aim from enhancing patient care, although the purposes and responsibilities may overlap. Just putting in place surveys of patient satisfaction establishes that the hospital is paying attention to the customer and to the customers' expectations. The information from surveys gives managers the insight that they need to 'see' and act on quality: it offers 'indicators' of areas for improvement (as we discuss later in the chapter).[12] This information supports the new textual surveillance of hospital work and its outcomes. So, while failing to consider much that was important to Hannah's care, patient satisfaction rankings stand in authoritatively for the actuality they claim to represent. Left out of the new account are the many aspects of poor patient care, sloppy handling of important information, poor and dangerous communication among professionals, and between family members and caregivers, as we have noted. If we take seriously what Janet and her aunt found from doing The Survey – for instance, that its structure largely prevented them from communicating what was important to them, that Hannah didn't know enough about what had actually happened to her to be a good witness, that they both tried but were often unsuccessful in making their meaning clear, then we need to think about what all this means for the hospital's management of quality of care. When a survey organizes patients' responses to their hospitalization, and reconstitutes them into levels of satisfaction, it organizes both what is accounted for in patient experiences, and just as important, *how that account is to be read*. Within the new public management's accounting logic, patients' expression of dissatisfaction would not necessarily be read for its *clinical* relevance. Managerial readers of the survey information have other things in mind besides the details of somebody's daily care being overlooked. Their attention must be focused on the 'big picture,' including the potentially serious issues of external visibility.

Hospitals are compared locally and nationally. Information from hospital patient satisfaction surveys provides a dataset 'whereby health-care organizations can assess their level of performance against a set of nationally applied standards' (Smith et al. 1999: 384). Hospital accreditation, now largely a textual review focused on the 'compliance' of local organizational practice with national standards (VCH News 2004), is itself conceptualized as quality improvement. Defining quality in 'terms of its dimensions or properties ... each [accreditation] criterion evaluated is linked to one of four quality dimensions: responsiveness, system competency, client/community focus and work-life' (CCHSA 2003 website). Patient satisfaction surveys, *whatever their ranking of satisfaction*, provide evidence of a hospital's systematic   client or customer focus, contributing thereby to the positive assessment of an institution's quality of care when one dimension is 'system competency.'

Besides formal accreditation, hospitals and health authorities are also attentive to how they are discussed in the media. Again, managers must be strategic. Patient satisfaction rankings have been given considerable public prominence recently. Popular magazines use Canadian Community Health Survey[13] data to reassure Canadians that 'despite polls that reveal the lowest ever public confidence in health care, surveys demonstrate that Canadians have consistently high levels of satisfaction with the health care they receive' (*Maclean's* 1999: 24). While acknowledging the usefulness of getting information out to the public, some researchers worry about this popularization of health information. The newsletter of the Canadian Health Services Research Foundation editorializes about the *Maclean's* ranking of the performance of health services, saying that 'the problem ... is that (the *Maclean's* rankings) would fail nearly every test of validity and reliability' (CHSRF 1999: 1–5). But media reports do not need to be overly attentive to academic niceties.

There is no question that the circulation of such information has a marketing function, apparently even for a not-for-profit organization. The literature suggests its relevance. For example, Gerteis et al. (1993: 242) say that 'patients who reported problems in (certain) areas ... were about four times more likely to say they would not return to that hospital in the future, and nearly nine times more likely not to recommend it to friends or families than those who did not experience such problems.' That similar concerns are now considered an issue in Canada is borne out by The Hospital's reporting that 'ninety percent of patients would prefer the same hospital if they were to require hospitalization again' and that 96% would recommend the hospital to their friends' (Summary Report 1995: 3). This reading of patient satisfaction information introduces into the Canadian context issues of patient (customer) loyalty as judged by potential referrals of family and friends, echoing the marketing framework of the 'for profit' system that Gerteis et al. write about. Canadian hospitals have reputations to uphold, and sometimes these are associated with important funding opportunities in which they are competitors.

Besides creating external visibility of an agency and its activities, patient satisfaction information has uses within the new data-driven techniques for exercising managerial control within health care settings. Just as the performance of provincial and regional health systems and hospitals are assessed comparatively, individual clinical practice units are also 'judged' through comparison of survey results. The rankings being created make not just the satisfaction of their patients (or of the staff) visible, but the information also speaks to the success of the respective unit managers. This new visibility inserts a competitive organizational approach into caregiving. In the patient-centred care literature, the work of the nursing unit manager is 'critical to performance' (Gerteis et al. 1993: 233). In The Hospital where Hannah was a patient, front-line nurse leaders, called clinical practice unit managers, were expected to make use of patient satisfaction ratings. As regards the 'overall care' rankings that are reported below, managers of psychiatry and orthopaedics units would have been expected to take some relevant action.

> With respect to the rating of Overall Care, 79% of patients rated the hospital as either 'Very Good' or 'Excellent' ... Differences among the Clinical Practice Units (CPUs) were seen with respect to patient satisfaction. Patients in the CPU of medicine were significantly more satisfied than patients in the CPU of psychiatry, and patients in the CPUs of Medicine and Surgery were significantly more satisfied than patients in the CPU of Orthopedics. (Summary Report 1995: 3)

Unit managers were expected to respond to trouble areas. It was still early days in the managerial use of satisfaction rankings when Rankin was collecting her ethnographic data. This may explain why the coordinator of hospital evaluation, whom she interviewed, felt that the 1998 survey data were 'underutilized.' However, the coordinator had plans for generating increased enthusiasm and compliance. Citing the expense and complexity of running the satisfaction surveys, she went on to say that 'in preparation for the next survey we have asked all the unit managers to sit on three committees that will involve them right from the planning stage; we are going to get their input in how to organize the data to make it [sic] useful for them; if we can get good buy-in from the start of the project they will be more invested to act on the data when we get it.'

This coordinator's need to get 'buy-in' and the strategies being developed to garner a more active responsiveness to the survey rankings among front-line nurse managers echo a similar theme, discussed in Chapter 3. 'Buy-in' is one of those ubiquitous concepts associated with successful implementation of managerial strategies that underscores that new values are being promoted, as well as new practices. Unit managers must learn to work on the basis of textual ways of knowing – the virtual reality of the new public management. A good deal of education goes into bringing nurse managers into this line of thinking.[14] Staff nurses, on the other hand, usually have to learn the approach in a less explicitly directed manner. The effects of the managerial strategies we have been describing – counting, comparing, standardizing, teaching, coaching, reporting, and so forth – often just appear in nurses' workplaces. When new information technologies arrive in their everyday work, nurses must pick up on how to '*know* the right things in the right way,' as they adapt themselves to nursing within a hospital operated on the basis of a virtual reality. This creates a new sort of tension for them. In the next chapter, we focus on nurses' learning and adapting to new priorities in health care.

For nursing managers, competitive attention to 'the best rankings' is relevant to their careers. To get ahead they must demonstrate compliance in addressing workplace problems as they are known textually. This helps to explain how it happens, at the same time, that direct knowledge of people's lives and experiences is subjugated. The amount of time available to attend to the day-to-day patient-care issues that arise is severely constrained. When a front-line nurse leader is engrossed within the relationships driven by the use of objectified information, that nurse leader's attention is diverted away from actual nurses, patients, and families. Not only is the information (about patient satisfaction, for instance) more objective and general than knowing from listening to a limited number of patients, but it is what 'counts' organizationally. It is processable, in ways that make it available for use by those in authority. These processes of ruling hook all members of the nursing staff into information processes, generating the virtual outcomes of 'quality,' 'efficiency,' 'productivity,' and so forth, by which the health care system's success is established.

The Critique of Nursing in Response to Virtual Accounts

In concluding this chapter we demonstrate the connection between knowing nursing as a virtual reality and knowing it as Janet and Hannah did. Returning to Janet's comments about the hospitalization, we want to bring forward, rather then suppress, her account of some of the problems experienced. It is our argument that some of these negative patient experiences have an organizational basis in the ruling practices of the new public management. We return, as well, to Dorothy Smith's 'actuality-data-theory' circuit because this formulation within the social organization of knowledge is key to our analysis. The Hospital experiences we describe have, in Smith's terms, been worked up through the 'ideological practice' (1990: 93) of hospital management: 'Ideological practices [are] methods of creating accounts of the world that treat it selectively in terms of a predetermined conceptual framework. The categories structuring data collection are already organized by a predetermined schema; the data produced become the reality intended by the schema; the schema interprets the data' (1990: 93–4).

This is an analytic description of what happens in the production and use of the virtual reality through which hospital settings are known authoritatively. With such systems of knowledge available for use, what nurses know about what happens on hospital units loses credibility. Now, more than ever, attention to the perspective of nurses recedes. Our next analytic step is to demonstrate how this is significant for nurses – and in this case, for patients, too.

Janet was convinced that Hannah's problems were exacerbated because there was no nurse whose job it was to maintain an overview of the nursing care, tracking and attending to the day-to-day concerns of patients and nurses. According to an interview Rankin conducted subsequently, any one of the nurses coming on duty for a shift might be assigned to be 'in charge.' The charge nurse would be responsible for such things as assigning nurses a specific workload of patients and monitoring the general condition of patients and the nursing response to all the patients on the unit. This is the vision of how self-directed, multiskilled nursing teams operate. Returning to Janet's observations and interactions with nurses, we recognize that the nurse with 'in charge' responsibilities was frequently unable to carry out any coordinating duties. In part, this is because nurses rotated constantly through the in-charge position and no one nurse had the opportunity to 'really know what is going on' (staff nurse interview) with patients and staff. Also, in addition to the responsibilities of being in charge, that nurse had her own group of patients to care for and constantly juggled the needs of the general ward nurses (and their patients) against her own work demands and those of the patients for whom she was personally responsible.

Some rather important trouble developed in Hannah's care. By reviewing the ethnographic accounts and considering the work organization in which they occurred, we can begin to see how knowing the setting ideologically might have influenced what happened. For instance, the accounting logic of patient-centred care would underpin and justify economies in nurse staffing that appeared to be a problem for Hannah's nursing care. The non-professional staff who handled Hannah's meals were not able to accurately assess and monitor Hannah's fluid balance when, on a tightly timed schedule, they delivered and picked up her meal trays. Janet was critical of what happened when there was no nurse who knew Hannah well enough to help individualize and properly contextualize her assessments and interventions while she was cared for by a constantly changing stream of casual (on-call) nurses. Hannah became constipated as a result of the painkillers she was taking, and that was overlooked for several days, perhaps owing to the 'efficient' organization of nurse staffing that abstracts patients into units of workload. Cost constraint might have been the reason that Hannah was frequently cared for by casually employed nurses. This seems to have affected her care adversely. For example, Hannah's intravenous access was not changed for seven days, at the end of which her arm had become reddened and painful. (The recommended standard for reviewing IV access is every three days.) Perhaps her (casual) nurses didn't take personal responsibility for Hannah's ongoing care, but were focused, instead, on accomplishing the work of just their own shift.[15] When Hannah experienced chest pain, there was no one available to respond to events in an individual way, no one who had been following Hannah's progress with whom the nurses could consult. Mistakes were made and even repeated. Given the needs of a contingent workforce, it appears that Hannah's nurses needed more direction than was available within the self-managed team. Could contingent staffing explain why, on almost every occasion, Hannah received hurried or standardized responses to her symptoms, ones that from the perspective of Janet's professional knowledge displayed marked inadequacies?

Janet saw how a focus on textual accounts and responsibilities displaced the front-line nurse leader's willingness or capacity to respond to patient and family experiences. Was it the nursing manager's shift to a text-mediated managerial job function that was played out in Janet's failed attempt to get help when Hannah's intake and output record was overlooked? The nursing manager whom Janet consulted about Hannah's excessive thirst tried to be helpful, but she was captivated by her managerial duties and priorities, and it became an 'administrative' concern about family access to documents. This illustrates how the front-line nurse leader is no longer embedded in the everyday world of nursing care, where nurses are busy and sometimes forgetful, where patients are thirsty and uncomfortable, and where family members make anxious appeals. The nursing manager must be attentive to problems that come to her in texts – in statistics and memos. These require that her attention be turned to entirely different kinds of issues.

Our analysis offers a glimpse not just into the problems that Janet described around Hannah's care, but into the organization of her care. These glimpses of the nursing setting are suggestive of an organization that 'creates a disjuncture between the world as it is known within the relations of ruling and the lived and experienced actualities its textual realities represent as 'what actually happened/what is' (Smith 1990a: 96). The taken-for-granted goodness of this new social organization is what we are criticizing. Besides the issue of professional hierarchies and related power, our analysis opens up the troubling issue of ideological accounts. We insist that the work of caring must include a consideration of what remains outside – discarded – by the ideological practices of knowing. These knowledge practices create a new hierarchy between those who theorize, formulate, conceptualize and make policy, and allocate resources and the front-line workers who remain in actual contact with patients. Our analysis of the Patient and Family Surveys supports Smith's observation that 'an organization can virtually invent the environment and objects corresponding to its accounting terminologies and practices' (1990a: 96). The organizational impregnability of such ideological circles has been identified elsewhere (Irvine et al. 1979). Supported by organizational hierarchy, and the power and domination accorded to new methods of governance and management, these forms of organizational knowing are sacrosanct.[16] In the next chapter, we explore how they draw nurses into the ideological circle.

6 Language and the Reorganization of Nurses' Consciousness

We have argued that health care reform takes place through text-mediated practices in which nurses are active participants. Various texts 'instruct' new nursing practices. Nurses engage in what we call text-reader conversations about what they might do for assigned patients (already constituted within the accounting logic of the new public management of health care reform.) In these text-reader conversations, the contemporary nursing workforce is learning new ways to practice nursing. As subjects in these text-mediated conversations, nurses act within their professionally approved and sanctioned capacities and become participants in a discourse that happens in sequences of social action (Smith 1999: 195).

Not just nursing work, but nurses themselves are changed in this process. Like Smith in *Writing the Social,* we too want to understand more about how people's, in this case nurses,' 'diversity of experience, perspective, and interest is coordinated into a unified frame at the institutional level' (1999: 195). This coordination is particularly relevant to the reform of health care, where the ideas, theories, commitments, and long-standing practices of individual health professionals are potentially destabilizing of the new public management agenda. Coordinating a managerial standpoint in a health care workplace has two major components: (1) the information infrastructure to which particular work processes are articulated, and (2) the engagement of the health care providers in activating the managerial project. In the latter, nurses themselves begin to think of health care as if its efficiency were their main business.

In previous chapters we have shown nurses encountering and activating the new information-oriented work processes in health care workplaces. Now we turn our attention to how nurses develop the capacity to engage as subjects in restructuring nursing. It has been argued elsewhere that engaging in textual practices that universalize or objectify what is known creates 'forms of consciousness that override the 'naturally' occurring diversity of perspectives and experiences' (Smith 1999: 195). It is this dominating effect on nurses' consciousnesses that we explore in this chapter. Our interest is in exploring how language helps, or might help, in 'sustaining the dominance of a particular standpoint as universal' (Smith 1990: 145). This piece of our inquiry draws on the thinking of several language theorists who direct our attention to understanding language and meaning as central to social organization. 'For these thinkers, meaning is always relational, processual, and *two-sided*,' according to Smith (1999: 142). For institutional ethnographers that two-sidedness or relational quality of speech and words can be explored 'for how [speech and words] coordinate or align individual consciousnesses, hence as *organization*' (ibid.). We turn to the nursing literature for 'exhibits' of how this can happen. We contend that these particular nurse writers have learned the accounting logic of the new public management, and their writing illustrates what we mean by nurses' consciousnesses being reorganized.

Double-sided Concepts, Speech Genres, and Spheres of Activity

Texts, instructions, and procedures of calculation, as well as of therapeutic action, constitute one side of nursing workplace restructuring, while nurses' – as well as other health practitioners' – reading, writing, hearing, thinking, and acting are the other side. To become organizationally competent, nurses, already competent in the nursing discourse, must learn how to work within organizational language. Consider, in this regard, the concept of 'quality of care.' It can be read as either a nursing or an organizational concept. In the situation reported earlier, where the Nurses United for Change actively pursued the troubles that they were experiencing in their work, it was their understanding of quality of care that energized them.[1] They recognized that quality of care was a concern shared by their administration and by the public. Given their hospital's quality assurance procedures, these nurses expected that their concerns about the quality of nursing care would be addressed when reported. Their reading of the quality assurance reporting process was that it meant *what they meant* by 'quality.' These nurses were unable or unwilling, at this point, to do an organizational reading. Thus, their interpretation of the situation (and of 'quality of care') was at odds with the institutional order being put in place and the virtual reality that was to define quality.

Excerpts from our field notes demonstrate the double-sidedness of the concept 'quality' and how the concept's two readings are part of different social relations. To illustrate, we offer here first a nursing and then an organizational reading. Rankin interviewed a nurse who was involved in the care of a woman who had undergone gynaecological surgery. The patient had been sent home and, inadvertently, had not had her vaginal packing removed. The nurse interviewed described how a home care nurse, visiting the patient some days later to address the woman's ongoing difficulties with urination, had discovered this serious oversight. From her own detailed recollections about the patient's urinary and catheter problems while in hospital, the nurse informant criticized the 'quality of nursing care' that the patient had received. In another instance, an organizational reading of the term 'quality of care' came to Rankin's attention when she interviewed one of The Hospital's patient care directors. This nursing manager referred to 'quality of nursing care' in discussing the average length of intensive care stay for patients who had suffered myocardial infarction (colloquially, a heart attack). This patient care director was not referring to a specific incident but identifying issues that she interpreted as quality of care in the unit's performance statistics over a six-month period and within the context of changes in the 'staffing mix.' It was her job to make sure that patients were cared for within the statistical guidelines that were being established as benchmarks across the region and further afield. Notice that both nurses were speaking from their work experiences, about their engagement in activities that related to the provision of quality of care.

Rankin, and almost anybody else who hears or reads the accounts made by the two nurses, could recognize them as 'making sense.' They did not only make sense syntactically; Rankin, a nurse herself, in conversation with each nurse, could fill out the content of the accounts sufficiently to recognize that they spoke competently. As used here, 'competence' relates to the speaker knowing and referring correctly to the relevant context of what she is talking about. This insider's capacity arises from the speaker's social location(s). Smith (1999) draws on Mead (1992), Bakhtin (1981, 1986), and Vološinov (1973) to argue that language is generated within social acts. In this case, the language of 'quality' could be said to be generated in each nurse's work. Behind these particular nurses' participation in 'utterances' – Bakhtin's word for speech and writing – are specific social and textually mediated practices of knowing 'quality of care.' Non-nurses are likely to fail to use words in the same way that people grounded in the activities of the settings do, revealing their location as outsiders to the work settings – and thus their lack of competence in the distinctive language use.

Smith (1999)[2] insists that the meaning of words arises from their situated usage rather than the other way round – where words 'simply symbolize a situation or object which is already there in advance' (Mead 1947, cited in Smith 1999: 114). This matters to our analysis because it suggests that we can trace language use back into social organization and into what Bakhtin (1986) calls particular 'spheres of activity' (1981: 60). Although each 'utterance' is individual, Bakhtin says that any sphere in which language is used 'develops its own *relatively stable types* of these utterances' that he refers to as 'speech genres' (ibid. 60). Speech genres 'bear the imprint of the characteristic usages associated with the activities of a group – a work organization, a professional practice, the experience of a generation, and the like' (Smith 1999: 120). 'The distinctive language uses that Bakhtin calls speech genres – terminology, syntactic conventions, stylistics, and so on – carry and regenerate the social organization of groups, large-scale organizations, and discourse, indeed, all forms of social life in which people together are concerting their activities in some specialized way' (Smith 1999: 143). This suggests why it is important for us to pay careful attention to how nurses use language and how their choice of language use comes about.

In the use of language reported above, the two nurses referred to something quite different when they spoke of quality of care. In light of the foregoing discussion, it becomes apparent that they were speaking from different locations within the health care setting and using the respective speech genres of each, where different knowledge and skills are required and exercised. One was a nurse giving direct care on a nursing ward. The other was a director of patient care, a nurse with management responsibilities. Their distinctive speech genres call up, at least for someone who is familiar with the settings, these different spheres of activity.

As we are illustrating, the nursing sphere is being changed, dominated by accounting logic through the use of text-mediated technologies of management. Nurses are learning to speak the language of those changes – a new form of engagement in their work. Language is central to the new forms of action. Smith argues that language or 'utterances' do not merely *express* social organization but they 'organize consciousnesses in courses of action' (1999: 145). The social relations of the organizational use of the terms 'quality' and 'quality of nursing care' project particular authoritative meanings into any situation that may exist in the work lives of nurses who care for patients. 'The social relations are not a context for the use of the term but the use of the term, how it means there, is part of the activity forming the relation' (Smith 1990b: 109). Given this understanding of language use, to discover the relations in which the different uses of the term 'quality' participate, we must explore the socially organized activities where they arise. Some instances have appeared in earlier chapters. Recall that it was an organizational description that informed and authorized how the nursing consultants at the NUC hospital could be 'impressed with the high quality of care provided' in the research hospital (External Nursing Review, 19 June 1996); this happened, even though the consultants heard the troubling stories collected by the NUC (including the story about a discharged patient's vaginal packing being overlooked). There, the organizational account superseded the experiential account. On occasion, the same term may be heard or read as being about the same thing (or, as Smith has said, words are 'a two-sided act'; 1999: 112). So, when 'quality of nursing care' finds objective expression in statistics, it is part of a sphere of activity distinct from nursing. Its meaning is different there from its meaning in the utterances of nurses, whose speech genre arises from the actualities of their work. Expressed in social acts, the concept 'quality' carries its meaning into various settings of use. It draws its users into that particular social organization. But even as the word is spoken by and acted on by nurses, its social organization remains implicit. To make language explicit and visible – and understandable as social organization – requires further analytic work.

Blended Speech Genres and Ruling Relations

Nurses encounter and interpret organizational texts and language in the routine process of considering what their job requires them to do (today, right now, first, and so on). Nurses are engaged knowledgeably in their work. Their knowing is central to their professional practice. Contemporary nursing is never simply procedural, the accomplishment of a list of tasks. Even a highly procedural nursing work process (such as that required by a clinical pathway) is always activated individually and knowledgeably, guided by the nurses' professional education. Nurses' education has prepared them to engage with abstract, conceptual language, 'building an intellectual bridge between nursing work and scientific knowledge' (Campbell 1995: 222). This capacity, it has been argued, was integral to establishing nursing 'as an academic discipline which requires [nursing] students to learn to think and do nursing in relation to abstract theories of nursing' that, according to Campbell (ibid.), informed curriculum changes in Canadian nursing beginning in the 1960s. On the basis of this kind of education and its subsequent evolution, nurses are expected to be able to theorize their choices for action – an intellectual and professional advancement over prior approaches to nursing.

The capacity to conceptualize nursing theoretically is also the basis for representing it in abstract language and textual form. This is a double-edged sword. As argued here, when texts mediate nursing action, the language used and its distinctive meaning arise from within some definite sphere of activity. The texts mediating nurses' work originate somewhere, not necessarily in nurses' own sphere of activity. Somebody makes up these organizational texts, and in the restructuring project, their origin would most likely have been outside the sphere of nursing. In this regard, think of the ADT and ALC texts, as examples. Our analysis in previous chapters has shown how activating these managerial texts draws nurses into extended social relations, into a practice of dominance.

Working with theoretical concepts has a similar organizing effect. Consider 'holistic care' and how front-line nurse leaders want the nurses to activate that concept (Chapter 4). We saw how an alternative speech genre, organized within its own sphere of activity, inserted an accounting logic and new ruling relations into nurses' work. When front-line nurse leaders want nurses to understand expeditious discharges as 'holistic' practice, nurses are expected to revise their nursing interpretation of 'holism' (already understood as the physical, emotional, social, economic and spiritual needs of a person), adding a new and expanded set of actions. The relation being established is between holism, as nurses know it from their nursing theory, and the hospital's discharge planning – specifically, the text of a 'social history' encountered in a restructured workplace. Being abstract, holism does not prescribe practical nursing activities. Nurses fill in what is unstated, making an assessment of and judgement about what the concept is calling for, and then they take the associated action. We used the example of a nurse acting to relieve an elderly hospital patient's worries about her dog, left unattended at home. Contrast this with hospital nursing before nurses were educated to work with the concepts of nursing theories, when patients' bodies and physical needs were the relevant object of nurses' work, and any activities related to patients' emotional or social needs were not theorized but understood as nurses' kindness or compassion (or lack thereof).

Our data show that the managerial goal of efficient discharge is also enlarging, and specifically shaping, nurses' sphere of attention and activity. Nurses already have resources on which they can draw to help them make such interpretations. They 'know' that people are more comfortable in their own homes than they are in the busy, impersonal, and institutional setting of the hospital. This idea has been popularized by the official studies of costs of health care conducted during the 1990s, including the one in British Columbia whose final report was called *Closer to Home* (1993). This report and others like it rationalize early discharge as being in the patient's best interests. Learning about the patient's home context, identifying available supports, and identifying barriers to the patient's ability to manage at home seem to fit with the nursing concept of holism. But let's rethink this. In our data, the *activity* that this so-called holistic practice is organizing is the completion of a standardized form; its purpose is to initiate an automatic referral – to social workers or community liaison nurses – of all newly admitted patients who meet certain pre-established criteria. This form-filling work, aimed at the managerial goal of expediting patient discharges, attends to management problems around pressure on available space and the hospital's productivity. Here the double-sided concept of holism as social acts blends nursing into the managerial sphere of activity. This is where a conflict arises for nurses. In this activity, the patient's best interests are not the issue and actually may be overlooked, as we have already seen. The new public management of the hospital has intervened between the concept of holism and nurses' interpretation and action. Holism, when the concept is used to call up activities that nurses would otherwise treat as outside their interest in caring for patients, exercises a regulating effect on nurses' consciousness, drawing them seamlessly into the restructuring project.

Holism, in this instance, is a word from one speech genre whose double meaning carries nurses over into another speech genre and into the social relations being constituted there. Smith has noted the 'organizing work [that] language will do,' and quoting Bakhtin (1981: 204), she draws attention to how words already exist 'in other people's mouths, in other people's contexts, serving other people's intentions' (1999: 142). That reflects exactly what we are seeing. In the situation we have been exploring, specific language is used for the purpose of organizing nurses' full and active participation in 'other people's intentions,' blending a sanctioned meaning from nursing with the different sphere of activity aimed at. The double meaning works as organization if, as managers count on, nurses accept as their own this new step in the work process. Our analysis emphasizes that, as in this example, language use is part of a ruling relation. Unless we hang on to that notion, it becomes impossible to see how nurses' work is being organized 'against them' – with all that that entails.

The Language of Efficiency and Reorganization of Nurses' Professionalism

Nurses understand that the pressures on the health care system are real and that the management technologies that they encounter, including those we have been describing, are in response to those pressures. Throughout the 1990s nurses, as well as other Canadians, heard and became widely accepting of the idea that the federal government's budget deficit justified cutbacks in health care funding.[3] These sorts of media-circulated messages hooked a variety of audiences, including nurses, into accepting and approving new measures for improving hospital efficiency. The restructuring of hospitals, what people speak about very non-specifically as 'change' and 'innovation' in the organization and delivery of health care, is widely held to be a good and reasonable thing. Nurses participate in this expression of public opinion. Beyond that, as we argue here, their involvement as actors and subjects in health care organizes their 'consciousnesses in courses of action' (Smith 1999: 145). As the speech genre of restructured health care becomes theirs, its accounting logic expressed in the language of efficiency becomes a central and familiar theme of nursing itself – so much so that the double-sided language of efficiency shapes nurses' understanding of restructuring as their own *professional responsibility*.

Nurses have always accepted the importance of being efficient in their work. As nursing students, they are taught to pay careful attention to how they coordinate their nursing activities so that they will make the best use of their time and energy. But the concept of efficiency evolves as the social practices that it names change. Janet Rankin offers her own experience of discovering how the efficiency she learned about in nursing school turned into a different concept of efficiency taught in nursing management classes in her post-RN degree program:

> In my own 1970s diploma nursing education I recall being told that my first priority was patient safety. Avoiding risk to patients was always to be foremost in my attentions and plans. Once safety was attended to, I was instructed to attend to patient suffering and to provide comfort. Finally, I was told, I was to attend to efficiency – the most practical way of accomplishing the work. I had to be organized, sequencing my tasks to use my energy sensibly to make sure I completed the required work in a reasonable amount of time. 'Safety, comfort and efficiency' became my organizing mantra (and likely the mantra of my nursing generation) for making nursing care decisions.

A decade later the language had taken on a new 'business-like' inflection. In 1984, when she was upgrading her professional credentials, a course on management was included in the core curriculum of Rankin's Bachelor of Science in Nursing program. Assigned readings framed efficiency quite differently from how she had previously understood it. One course text put it this way:

> Efficiency is a vital part of management. It refers to the relationship between inputs and outputs. If you get more output for any given input, you have increased efficiency. Similarly, if you can get the same output from less input you again increase efficiency. Since managers deal with input resources that are scarce – money, people, and equipment – they are concerned with the efficient use of these resources. Management therefore is concerned with minimizing resource costs. It is not enough to be merely efficient. Management is also concerned with getting activities completed; that is, it seeks effectiveness. When managers achieve their organization's goals, we say they are effective. So efficiency is concerned with means and effectiveness with ends. (Robbins 1984: 5)

In the above excerpt, nurse-readers are offered an interpretive schema of efficiency that represents managerial interests. Within this framework, Janet and other nursing students were introduced to the conceptual tools that they would use to activate efficiency in a different way. 'Formerly,' said Janet, 'my responsibility for efficiency related to my own skills – my individual clinical judgment, priority-setting, and time management were at the centre of that form of efficiency. Now I was being involved in an efficiency that encompassed broader organizational considerations, in which I was being prepared to participate, in various ways.' In a later text, Robbins and co-author Langton demonstrate the salience of efficiency for other sites of public service and explicitly develop the concept of efficiency (within what we are now calling the new public management orientation) when they explain that 'a hospital, for example, is effective when it successfully meets the needs of its clientele. It is efficient when it can do so at a low cost. If a hospital manages to achieve higher output from its present staff – say, by reducing the average number of days a patient is confined to a bed, or by increasing the number of staff-patient contacts per day – we say the hospital has gained productive efficiency' (2003: 11).

In this text, health care is being thought about in a new way. The authors include Canadian health care explicitly and unproblematically as a site for improved productivity 'in order to make our goods and services competitive in the global market' (2003: 12).

The evolving meaning of efficiency is carried through the burgeoning field of nursing management (e.g., Branowicki and Shermont 1997; Hibberd and Smith 1999) and finds its way into the mouths of nurses doing direct practice. It gains a practical foothold in the sphere of nursing activity as it is written into the new job descriptions of front-line nurse leaders (Chapter 4). It guides nurses to conceptualize their activities as 'inputs' and patients as 'outputs,' and promotes a nursing interest in doing 'more for less.' It appears in the organizational activities of measurement, calculation, comparison,and competition, as nurses learn that success is expressed in virtual realities. We have described (in Chapter 3) how we found an explanation about 'efficient use of resources' justifying Nurse Trudy's discharge of a confused and incontinent postoperative patient into the care of his wife, possibly jeopardizing the safety of both partners. Nurse Linda (in Chapter 2) was organized by efficiency measures when she contravened the mandate to attend to her patient's comfort and discharged a decidedly nauseated patient without appropriate treatment. While these nurses may have recognized that their nursing care was not optimal, they accepted as their priority the optimizing of the use of hospital resources.

Nurses' competent use of the language of efficiency identifies, for us, the double relation of which nurses are becoming a part. On the one hand, nurses retain their traditional understanding of their responsibility to be efficient. Their work with patients in busy hospitals requires them to be well organized if they are to identify and attend to individual needs. On the other hand, the accounting logic of the concept as it now circulates in the discourse dominates their thinking and influences how they act. Nurses, like Linda and Trudy, are learning to take seriously their own responsibility to act in ways that accommodate and advance a hospital's cost savings. This requires a shift in their consciousness. We recognize a number of ways in which that happens, including through the professional discourse of nursing.

As early as 1992 articles appeared in nursing journals reflecting nurses' naturalization of the blended concept of efficiency. In one such article Canadian nurses Sandhu, Duquette, and Kérouac[4] (1992) assert the necessity of adapting nursing practices to the reductions in health-care funding. These nurse-authors implicitly accept that the funding cuts are necessary, too. Noting that 'nursing administrators are desperately looking for a means of reducing costs of care in institutions,' they indicate how 'nursing care has to be congruent with the expectations of societies in the 1990s' (1992: 33). The particular contribution that these writers make is to suggest a 'managed care' strategy in which 'the care is geared towards reducing the number of hospital days for a patient' (ibid.). Efficiency-oriented assignment patterns (achieving altered nurse-patient ratios) make sense to them, and to their readers, within this framework. 'These times of cost constraint' is normalized or naturalized as 'how things are.' That being so, the background out of which the necessity springs needs no analytic attention. Nurses are able to see and accept cost constraint and the restructuring of their work as common sense. Roxana Ng (1995) writes of similar situations that she has puzzled over where commonsensical explanations seem to replace any need to analyse what is actually going on. She explains what she sees as the operation of an 'ideological frame' of multiculturalism that, once in place, 'renders the very work processes that produced it invisible, and the idea it references as "common sense" ... and taken for granted as "that's how it is" or "that's how it should be"' (1995: 36).

As Ng suggests (regarding her own context), the work processes that produce nursing's blended concept of efficiency and that point to *its necessity* have become almost invisible. It is even difficult to think about 'work processes' producing what we otherwise 'know' and accept as true about efficiency. Such practices are becoming taken for granted as aspects of contemporary nursing. But if we look carefully,

we can 'find' the processes that produce an invisible ideological framework in the nursing discourse. For instance, the writing of Sandhu et
al. creates discursively organized subject positions 'congruent with the
expectations of societies in the 1990s.' As we read, we find ourselves
adopting the standpoint of their text. Doing so positions readers (us) to
see the point that these nurses make. From that position in the text,
what they say makes sense to readers. Nurses reading articles such as
the one by Sandhu et al. (1992) will enter into their particular interpretive framing of their everyday experience and see in it 'the necessity' of
the efficiency project.

   We now turn to an examination of how nurses' writing establishes
'subject positions in the discourse' for themselves and other nurses. We
argue, following Smith (1999: 94), that from such discursively organized subject positions 'experience can be known only externally and
from within an order of domination.' Such a reading encourages
nurses to reinterpret their experience, revising it and forgetting their
local history. Their standpoint in their everyday world of nursing (and
their knowing from it) is subdued. In two analytic exhibits,[5] using texts
from the nursing discourse that came readily to hand, we explore these
claims. The first article that we examine was published in the *Canadian
Nurse*, a professional journal to which nurses are automatically sub-
scribed when they register to practise nursing in Canada. The second is
an article from the *Journal of Family Nursing* that Rankin assigns to be
read by her class of second-year nursing students. Our analysis focuses
on the language that the writers use to 'come to terms' with contemporary nursing problems. We show, in these exhibits, nurse writers fully
engaged as subjects, identifying issues of serious concern to them and
other nurses. Our aim is not simply to criticize what they say. Indeed,
in reading these pieces, we find ourselves being persuaded by their
arguments. Our analytic purpose is to figure out and exhibit how the
writing works to successfully engage us in these authors' thinking,
their point of view, their account of 'the trouble,' and their proposed
solutions. We, of course, use our own analytic framework and our
interest in language to account for and respond to their arguments.

**'A surgical liaison nurse embraces the family as part of the
continuum of care and promotes holistic nursing practice'[6]**

An article by three nurses (Fowlie, Francis, and Russell 2000) who are
employed in nursing management positions describes a solution to a pervasive problem within their hospital. The article's banner states (2008: 30):

1-01 In one Halifax hospital, a surgical liaison nurse embraces the family
1-02 as part of the continuum of care and promotes
1-03 holistic nursing practice.

As part of a quality improvement project, a new nursing position called a surgical liaison nurse (SLN) has been created and evaluated. This article is in the form of a short project report. Ostensibly writing about 'family nursing,' 'holistic practice,' and a 'continuum of care,' the authors 'utter' the new conjoined language genre (nursing and management). Immediately after the article's banner (1-01 to 1-03), the SLN is said to provide a 'communication link' informing and supporting patients and families before, during, and after surgery. 'Communication *problems*' is the blended concept that the writers were able to produce as a convincing interpretive framework for a litany of troubles in the hospital. As early as line 1-04 to 1-06, they write:

1-04 We recognized that in the growing same-day-admit and day-surgery
1-05 programs there was a lack of communication between the
1-06 perioperative team and families.

For the authors, the initiative to improve communication solved the problem of regular nursing staff not having time to talk to the families of patients undergoing surgery in the new 'efficient' day-surgery program. Examples given of troubles occurring in the hospital settings include the following (2000: 31):

1-07 Family members were often left alone for hours with no information
1-08 about the patient. As a result they would stop any professional
1-09 they saw in the hallways for information.
1-10 Families were both concerned and frustrated because
1-11 they did not know what was happening during the operation.
1-12 Anesthetists and nurses transporting patients to the post-anaesthetic
1-13 care unit had to make their way around the worried family members
1-14 of other patients in the hallways. When uninformed family members
1-15 went to the post-recovery lounge to enquire about the patient, the
1-16 same-day-admit staff interrupted their nursing care of other patients
1-17 to meet the families' needs.

Nurse-readers will understand and empathize with families' worries, concerns, and frustrations. But as quickly as line 1-16, they are offered a different interpretation, blending such traditional nursing concerns about worried families into the framework of efficiency. Concern about family members' frustrations and worries is painted over a commanding backdrop that offers competent nurse-readers the concept of *interruptions* to the smooth rolling out of the ambulatory surgical program. To understand the importance to nurses of interruptions, we need to recall (from Chapter 2) Windle's (1994) description of clinical pathways for postanaesthetic recovery. In the clinical pathway to which she refers, the patient's hospital stay is divided into half-hour intervals, and nursing intervention is directed – textually – minute by minute. Nurse-readers who have firsthand knowledge of the rationalized use of time in restructured hospitals will easily recognize how interruptions are a problem. They will know that when families 'stop any professional they saw in the hallways for information' (1-08–09), or when 'nurses transporting patients to the post-anaesthetic care unit had to make their way around the worried family members of other patients in the hallways' (1-12–14), or when the 'same-day-admit staff interrupted their nursing care of other patients to meet the families' needs' (1-16–17) that precious nursing time is *wasted*. We can assume that the subject position established in the discourse is easily adopted by nurse-readers who have had such experiences.

For us, and other readers who are nurses or who have been family members of patients it is immediately apparent that there are potential benefits to be gained from the project that these authors report. Reading as health professionals, nurses will find echoes of their own everyday experience. For those reading as family members of a hospitalized patient, the language calls up similar experiences of waiting, not knowing what to expect – (recall from a previous chapter where Janet felt far from 'embraced' as she navigated the hospitalization of her head-injured aunt). The Halifax initiative seems to offer something for everybody. Intended for nurses, it offers a way around the problems that families create for *them*. Readers who have similar experiences to Janet's with the contemporary Canadian health care system will be optimistic that this kind of initiative might meet their needs.

What this reading (either as a nurse and a family member) drops away is the restructured context in which this new role for a perioperative nurse makes sense. Early in the article, the authors write enthusiastically about the broad scope of the surgical program which, through regionalization, is being administered over two hospital sites. The overall reduction of length of stay (LOS) of patients in Canadian hospitals – a key goal in restructuring – has been accomplished through same-day admit and day-surgery programs.[7] Fowlie et al. explain how the same-day-admit and day-surgeries account for '85–95% of the surgeries done' at their hospital (2000: 30). The authors of the Halifax report can rely on their nurse-readers not only to recognize and understand the programs that they refer to but to accept them as one of the major 'improvements' in hospital care that improve efficiencies, reduce costs, and shorten waiting lists.

Their article positions readers *not to see* the efficiency-oriented same-day surgical programs as other than successful and taken-for-granted accomplishments of quality improvement in hospital care. How does it do that? We argue that its success is in the use of the two speech genres that so convincingly blend the two spheres of activity in which nurses participate. Fowlie et al. focus their readers' attention on nurses' venerable interests – in patients' and families' comfort, reframed here as issues of communication. This interpretation positions readers to see how interruptions by families that interfere with the tightly organized movement of patients in and out of ambulatory care, portrayed here as poor nurse/family communication, could be avoided. That the new practices of the same-day-admit and day-surgery *create* the problems for nursing (and for families) does not surface in this perspective. The programs themselves are a 'given,' their effect being to improve the hospital's efficiency. To buttress this view, the writers use the discourse of quality improvement and celebrate the programs' success, for instance, by listing the awards their particular initiative achieved (2000: 33). Being applauded in the article is the creativity shown by nurses who developed new roles patching up the holes that restructuring has punched in nursing. For these nurses, the growth of ambulatory care programs that minutely direct nurses' time and attention is naturalized. (Here we see the cost of this restructuring to families; elsewhere we have shown other losses.) Yet this is what nurses know to be the everyday/everynight context of efficient practice.

Describing the (new) role of the surgical liaison nurse, Fowlie et al. (2000: 30) say that it

1-18 was developed as a quality improvement initiative with the
1-19 intent of providing a communication support and comfort link with
1-20 families of surgical patients.

Through substituting the discourse of quality improvement for nurses' interpretive framework, the article submerges the practical challenges that nurses face in the same-day surgical setting. The nursing language in the report draws us in. In the traditional speech genre of nursing 'lack of communication between the perioperative team and families' (1-05–06) and 'families were both concerned and frustrated' (1-10) encourages nurse-readers to focus on the needs and care of patients and their families. The double relation of the term 'quality' (1-18) provides a crossover link between nurses and managers. When aligned with words such as 'comfort link' and 'communication support,' quality seems to be what nurses know it to be. It seems a far cry from that to the accounting logic of a quality improvement program that aims at efficiency by boosting the productivity of surgical programs.

The continuing growth and promotion of cost-oriented efficiencies converge with nurses' established interests through language that refer to 'embracing the family as part of the continuum of care to promote holistic nursing practice' (1-01 and 1-02). The endorsements (1-21 to 1-26, below), gathered through family and staff surveys, are another way that Fowlie et al. (as co-actors in the quality improvement initiative) authorize readers to overlook the fundamentally negative impact that restructuring has on patients and staff.

1-21 'Finally, in our world of cutbacks there is a role that truly benefits the family.'

1-22 'I have witnessed on numerous occasions a sigh of relief when family members are informed that someone will be available to touch base with them.'

1-23 'What a comfort to have someone to answer questions and reassure me that all was going well.'

1-24 'Programs such as these should be enhanced and maintained. Personal contact and dialogue are sadly lacking in health care these days.'

1-25 'Information has a calming effect on family members.'

These comments of gratitude and relief expressed by family members and/or hospital staff highlight that the SLN role helped to plug the hole that 'our world of cutbacks' creates, while not noticing the hole, itself. In these comments, both positive and negative experience are available to be glimpsed. But we read the story positively. Nurse-readers are enrolled in translating their similar, including similarly negative, experiences into excitement about the possibilities that the new initiative offers. From subject positions created within the discourse, nurse-readers' experience of both their own and their patients' and families' troubles are interpreted 'only externally and from within an order of domination' (Smith 1999: 94). A competent reading of the following lines positions the reader for an interpretation that carries a dominant perspective.

1-26 'The person in this position [the surgical liaison nurse] has an incredible opportunity to make a real difference for the people's experience. It is a highly educational role, but offers a supportive caring face to what can be an isolating experience.'

The competent reader will interpret her own experience from the *external* position of quality improvement (the 'incredible opportunity,' 1-26). Recessive in this text are the 'isolating experience' (1-26) and the conditions that create it as well as the interventions 'sadly lacking' (1-25) in personal contact. As readers, we are positioned to understand it to be a good thing that family members who are calmed (1-25) will stay out of the way of the busy workers. We are positioned by the standpoint of the discourse that we adopt to respond hopefully to the sense making practices of the new public management.

This writing contributes to a discourse that, like the speech genres of the workplace, is blended. When one word reconciles two meanings and two spheres of activity, the conjoined language use helps create a fit between nurses' traditional interests and their new efficiency practices. These writers' competent use of blended language suggests that their own consciousness has been reorganized so that they have adopted as their own an efficiency-oriented version of proficient nursing. Although we as analysts insist that the fit between this sleight of language and nurses' traditional interests is illusory, the blending erodes nurses' capacity to speak from a standpoint in the everyday world of their work. And that attenuates nurses' grounds for challenging and resisting the disappearance of their own nursing interests from health care.

'Maximizing time, minimizing suffering: The 15-minute (or less) family interview'[8]

Lorraine Wright and Maureen Leahey are engaged in another kind of problem-solving to improve the practice of nursing in restructured workplaces. At one level of reading, their article and the one by Fowlie et al. are about the same thing – both address problems arising in health care when nurses are overly pressured. Wright and Leahey (1999: 260) say:

2-01 Time is of the essence in nursing practice. Major changes in the
2-02 delivery of health care services through budgetary constraints and
2-03 staff cutbacks have required new ideas for involving families.
2-04 Rather than excluding family members from health care, more efficient
2-05 ways need to be determined of how to conduct brief family
2-06 interviews.

Yet the differences between the two articles could hardly be more striking. They describe and promote different approaches, finding radically different solutions to virtually 'the same' problem. The writing arises from differently located spheres of activity. Fowlie et al. report briefly and objectively on the procedures that they used and the outcomes that they achieved in their carefully defined (managerial) project. The Wright and Leahey piece is longer, and being more academic, it makes reference to nursing theory; yet it is intensely practical and written in a style that is experiential and, at times, personal. Wright and Leahey offer a set of instructions for how nurses should conduct themselves when they think that they don't have time to talk to families – what the authros call nurses' 'constraining beliefs.'

2-07 Uncovering these constraining beliefs makes it more comprehen-
2-08 sible why nurses might shy away from routinely involving families in
2-09 nursing practice. We postulate that if nurses were to embrace only
2-10 one belief that 'illness is a family affair' (Wright et al. 1996: 288),
2-11 it would change the face of nursing practice.

According to these family nursing practitioners, who are also academics affiliated with the University of Calgary, nurses must use whatever opportunities they can find to involve themselves therapeutically with families and in that way 'alleviate and diminish suffering' (1999: 261).

This second article lays out, and then gives experiential examples, of what Wright and Leahey consider to be the key ingredients for including patients' families in brief therapeutic interaction. These include: (1) use of good manners, which, as they describe it, is a specific presentation of self by the nurse that 'instils trust' (1999: 263); (2) therapeutic conversations to give and acquire information relevant to care and that communicate the nurse's personal interest and understanding; (3) certain technical procedures for mapping a patient's family and other social supports; (4) instructions for the specific form of talk that nurses should use to accomplish therapeutic goals, for example, questions; and (5) 'commendations' (1999: 267) that elicit the collaboration of the patient and family and identify otherwise invisible needs that might undermine recovery and efficient discharge.

The picture of nurses that Wright and Leahey's writing creates is of capable and caring professionals, who accept both a moral and a strategic professional duty to interact therapeutically with patients and their families, even under difficult conditions. They present nurses as fallible, which suggests that nurses have another duty, as well – to improve themselves and their capacities.

We (Rankin and Campbell) find ourselves being convinced by this. As readers, we could and did take up this perspective, adopting the subject position being created in the text, through which the article is to be read. But we are reminded of Smith's (1999) claim that from a discursively organized subject position we can know experience only externally and from within an order of domination. Smith had been analysing the place of theory in sociological reading and writing. She was identifying the magisterial framing of an account (of experience) by theory. How would the Wright and Leahey text constitute within it a form of domination of one's reading? A hint about this comes from Wright and Leahey's own data about nurses' constraining beliefs that they 'have discovered' (1999: 260):

2-12 Some of these beliefs are: 'If I talk to family members I
2-13 won't have time to complete my other nursing responsibilities'; 'If I
2-14 talk to family members, I may open up a can of worms and I will
2-15 have not time to deal with it'; 'It's not my job to talk with families,
2-16 that's for social workers and psychologists'; 'I can't possibly help
2-17 families in the brief time I will be caring for them.'

While in the article 'staff cutbacks and budgetary restraints' are not ignored (2-02 and 2-03), Wright and Leahey insist that nurses' avoidance of family members results from their 'constraining beliefs' (2-07). They list what nurses with whom they interact in classes and professional workshops say about their experience of contemporary nursing. The nurses they quote speak of their experience of working in restructured workplaces. Treating the social organization of nurses' work as a taken-for-granted condition allows Wright and Leahey to propose that nurses need to develop new, 'more efficient' strategies (2-04). It occurs to us that downplaying the actual conditions within which nursing is done helps to create the illusion that nurses can maintain an unchanged quality of nursing service, if only they would change their beliefs and practices.

Wright and Leahey insist that what they expect of nurses is possible, and they give examples to prove it (1999: 270). They sum up a poignant vignette of Wright's own personal experience where 'in that one sentence, this nurse assessed and acknowledged my suffering [providing] comfort and understanding through her very brief interaction with me … This nurse demonstrated that family nursing can be done in busy emergency units, even in 2 minutes, and effect healing' (1999: 270). Theirs is the magisterial voice. The voices of the nurses in their data who 'don't have time' are isolated, decontextualized, and as such, they can be dismissed as wrong. Perhaps they are. We wouldn't actually know from this article. What we do know is that the focus on changing nurses' beliefs and behaviour, as a solution to lack of time, drops the social organization of their work out of sight. The organizing features of the actual work with family members that is being done by nurses (in restructured settings) are glossed over as nurses' 'constraining beliefs.'

As readers, we are persuaded, but as analysts, we are not. We cannot be, as long as we have a competing experiential account. It is crucial to note that the standpoint constructed in the Wright and Leahey text subjugates the standpoint of the nurses. When they use nurses' talk, the text frames what nurses say in ways that accomplish the authors' meanings. We contrast that with what we have tried to do in 'taking the standpoint of nurses' and exploring how their own talk about experiences and the experiences themselves are organized. In previous chapters we have offered instances of how interactions between nurses and families are actually organized, outside the nurses' beliefs, outside their intentions. Recall (in Chapter 3) how Nurse Trudy explained her discharge practices: 'She [the patient's wife] arrives and I introduce myself and I'm trying to figure out who she has already talked to, and I'm trying to slow down so that I can give her all this information in a way that won't be too overwhelming, I am rushing though, through the discharge instructions, the prescriptions, his bowel meds and stuff. So I'm talking to her, explaining about his incontinence and telling her where she can buy Attends [adult diapers].'

We are convinced that Wright and Leahey have something important to say to nurses such as Trudy. Their instructions for conducting brief encounters seem sound and indeed, helpful. But Trudy (and nurses like her) has something to show them, too. Trudy's time is not her own. Nurse Trudy did not need Wright and Leahey to point out that her patient's wife was 'influenced by and reciprocally influenced the illness' (2-25 to 2-26), and certainly, she did not need to be encouraged to be 'brief.' Two minutes would have been a very long time for Trudy when, under pressure, she had to accomplish a number of things that were time-relevant. In Trudy's everyday/everynight experiences, the material features of her work produced the 'brief family interview' that she conducted. Her use of her scarce time includes activating the increasing responsibility of unpaid family caregivers on which hospitals rely heavily to increase their efficiency and productivity. The material features of what actually happens between nurses and patients, such as Trudy's ad hoc advice to purchase adult diapers and the attempt to 'put in more home supports,' would not be visible in the accounts that Wright and Leahey make of nursing talk (and beliefs). They would not have approved of Trudy's interaction with a tearful and overburdened, and aging, family member. Trudy was not happy with it either. However, the restructuring of hospital practices created the conditions within which Trudy's options were narrowed. How she worked was sanctioned as efficient practice – just the way it happened. In that context, changing a nurse's practice involves more than Wright and Leahey seem to suggest.

2-18 For nurses' behaviors to change, they must first alter or modify
2-19 their beliefs about involving family members in health care.

As we consider our data and the stories we collected of nurses struggling to do their jobs well, we see a troubling disconnection between Wright and Leahey's focus on nurses' beliefs and the social organization of restructured hospitals. And that is what allows Wright and Leahey to expect significantly improved outcomes from changing nurses' beliefs.

2-20 Nurses would then be more eager to know how to involve and
2-21 assist family members in the care of their loved one. They would
2-22 appreciate that everyone in a family experiences an illness and
2-23 that no one family member 'has' diabetes, multiple sclerosis, or cancer.
2-24 By embracing this belief, they would realize that from initial onset
2-25 of symptoms, through diagnosis and treatment, all family members
2-26 are influenced by and reciprocally influenced the illness. They also
2-27 would come to experience how our privileged conversations with
2-28 patients and their families about their illness experiences can
2-29 contribute dramatically to healing and the diminishing or alleviation
2-30 of suffering.

These expectations, stripped of organizational context, now begin to appear as a form of domination in nurses' lives. Although 'disappeared' in the text, the ruling relations remain an organizing feature of the everyday/everynight workplace, trapping nurses. The text of the article makes invisible those socially organized relations of the nursing workplace. It is only when the actualities of nursing in the everyday/everynight world are dismissed that nurses' beliefs can be treated as what is wrong and what can and must be changed. The text creates a discursively organized standpoint in which nurses come to be responsible for successful therapeutic behaviour, no matter how their work is organized.

Our inquiry in this chapter has focused on nurses' language and the importance of specific language use in the professional nursing discourses. We have exhibited how language use organizes a particular standpoint, dominating nurse-readers' interpretations and, in a sense, disenfranchising nurses who would speak about what is actually happening to patient care. In this book we have been tying together an account of restructuring that reveals nurses 'competent' participation. They respond, as they must, to its ruling effects. Language use seems pivotal to nurses' engagement in restructuring their own practice. With Bakhtin, we have been interested in how language changes over time, but always maintaining its connection to related social changes. Bakhtin says: 'In order to puzzle out the complex historical dynamics of these systems [of language] and move from a simple (and, in the majority of cases superficial) description of styles, which are always in evidence and alternating with one another, to a historical explanation of these changes, one must develop a special history of speech genres that reflects more directly, clearly, and flexibly, *all the changes taking place in social life*. Utterances and their types, that is, speech genres, are the drive belts from the history of society to the history of language' (1986: 65, emphasis added).

The social life of nursing practice is being restructured. Within the historicity of that social restructuring, accomplished through the implementation of the new public management's efficiency practices, nursing discourse is also being restructured. A new speech genre is evolving. In this new speech genre, hospital and nursing managers adopt terms from the conceptual jurisdiction of the traditional professional nursing genre, and nurses adopt terms from the genre of hospital management. The altruistic language of nurses used by the nurse-writers we quoted are examples – 'embraces the family' (1-01), 'continuum of care' (1-02), 'holistic nursing' (1-03); 'meet the families' needs' (1-17), 'communication support and comfort link' (1-19), 'make a real difference' (1-26), 'illness is a family affair' (2-10), 'change the face of nursing' (2-11), 'privileged conversations' (2-27), 'contribute dramatically to healing' (2-29), and 'alleviation of suffering' (2-30) – this language provides the syntactical links that help to tie nurses, emotionally and intellectually, and as we argue here, professionally, to blended practices. A language is being developed that managers and nurses share. Its use carries with it and partakes in the ruling relation of hospital restructuring's accounting logic. Nurses fluent in the commonsensical shibboleths that 'Canadians need to live within their means' and that we can 'no longer afford our extravagant health and social spending' will easily buy into the new speech genre.

What emerges are disquieting contradictions within contemporary nursing. The profession increasingly speaks the language of restructuring as its own language. Nurses promote efficiency (and its priorizing of the economy, trade, and capital accumulation over the human and collective values of citizens) as a professional value. Of course, nurses living in the everyday/everynight world of health care recognize that efficiency practices have their own costs, creating troubles and disrupting nursing. And as we have shown, a range of negative consequences is not ignored by the profession and its leaders. Rather, from within a framework of domination, such problems become something (more) to be managed by nurses. Nurses who are fluent in the blended speech genre take up the task of managing nursing's new troubles. When they do, they become part of the ruling effort that dominates nurses. Nurses competent in organizational discourse continue to 'read past' the socially organized conditions of health care reform that account for the negative impacts on themselves and their colleagues, their practice, and their patients.

Conclusion

Across Canada nurses report for duty in health care institutions where, around the clock, their work coordinates and maintains the always contingent and unpredictable environment in which care takes place. Their knowledge and skills have long been relied upon to ensure that, not just nursing, but all the care of hospitalized patients unfolds safely, properly (and efficiently). Patients, families, physicians, and many allied health care workers trust nurses to know what is required, what to do, what must be done first, and what must be left out or done differently. In particular, nurses see to it that patients are prepared and available for treatment, given treatments on time, and observed for their response to treatment and that any difficulties are untangled so that corrective interventions can be made promptly. Much of nurses' work, like domestic work, takes place in the background, unaccounted for in formal job descriptions. But without it, knots would appear in the smooth rolling out of the collective endeavour that is hospital care.

As health care is reformed, nurses are expected to provide nursing care as usual. *Or do they* – provide care 'as usual'? It is around this issue of *how* nurses are involved in reformed institutions, therapeutic programs, and methods of administration that our inquiry has focused. In exploring several sites of nursing care ethnographically, we have pointed to changes that, as a result of health care reform and hospital restructuring, are reordering nurses' work. In stories about nurses Linda, Trudy, and Sara and patients Ms Shoulder, Mr and Mrs Jones, and Aunt Hannah, analysis of nursing activities directed us to the corresponding work of patient placement clerks, team leaders, hospital administrators, and health ministry bureaucrats. We have shown how knowing a health care setting, or even a patient, through a particular perspective (for instance, ruled by considerations of efficiency) remakes that setting or that patient. In so doing, it also remakes nursing. Our analysis opens up many apparent contradictions.

Despite assertions that health care reform and hospital restructuring are expected to improve nursing care (or at least leave it unfettered,[1] making it more patient-centred and socially relevant), we have shown nurses' work with patients being reformed in troubling ways. Many nurses accept the current requirement to develop more efficient ways to nurse patients and to act within the organization's restructuring mandate. Even those nurses who have not yet adopted the imperative for efficiency as their own are being captured within the new practices that this imperative organizes. No matter what they think, nurses themselves are agents of practices that disrupt their traditional standpoint. An unacknowledged gap opens as their work articulates patients and their needs to decisions made objectively within a reformed system that has been redesigned to know patients and their needs as numbers and categories. Even so, the everyday/everynight world remains unsubdued, not seamlessly consistent with accounts of it that nurses help to make.[2] This adds another challenge. Nurses are enacting policies made elsewhere, and they must reconfigure their activities to try to bring the actualities of their work into line with the accounting logic of the new public management. This is both a trap and an opportunity for nurses, as we shall explain.

New ways of knowing have entered the sphere of nursing work throughout the decades of health care reform and hospital restructuring. What nurses know from their everyday/everynight work is often at odds with their new, discursively organized, efficiency-oriented knowledge. We heard many stories of ordinary nursing care gone awry. Many of the nurses we spoke with questioned their ability to give 'good care' under the new systems. Nurses said that they were noticing more mistakes. According to them, instances of early signs and symptoms of complications such as infection, deep vein thrombosis, compartment syndrome, delirium, and so on, which would normally incite action, are now being overlooked. Nurses described their frustrations arising in the organizational efforts to make every penny count and saw the cost to them and their patients of the restructuring practices. Regarding bed utilization policies, for instance, they criticized 'back transfers' – moving patients from their beds on wards back to the Emergency Department in the middle of the night to accommodate postoperative trauma patients who had come in as emergencies.

Likewise, nurse informants complained of the disruption associated with playing 'musical beds' when patients are juggled from room to room and bed to bed among private, semiprivate, and isolation rooms to 'make a bed.' They described how their caring work has been infiltrated by numerous efficiency-oriented interruptions that distract them and leave them vulnerable to making mistakes. More experienced nurses, especially, talked about what it means when 'basic care' is no longer attended to. They worry that as bathing, mouth care, looking after dentures, shaving men's beards, attending to patient's bowel routines, and even the regular changing of bed linens are overlooked, it is forgotten that this care contributes to a patient's health and comfort and supports recovery. The move to knowing patients in a strictly scientific and objective way leads to less attention to (and less time available for) treating patients as people with needs beyond what is objectively measurable.

Missing what is important to nurses may have consequences for the very goals that reform emphasizes. Nurses suggest, for instance, that the basic elements underlying the efficiency of their own work are being overlooked, as efficiency is conceptualized by distant others and cast into commensurable terms. Some complain that they must work around chronic shortages of supplies and equipment. Tight control over the use of resources might seem sensible to cost accountants, but in the everyday/everynight world of nursing it is wasteful of nurses' scarce time and effort to be running to another floor to borrow equipment or linen. Nurses say that they are also experiencing diminishing support from other hospital departments (for example, housekeeping, dietary, maintenance, laundry, and pharmacy) in the new, more competitive, organizational environment. When everyone is anxiously watching their bottom line, they forget that the ultimate goal of all their work is patient care. We saw indications of all this in our participant observations of nurses at work. We observed nurses adapting, making do, cutting corners, and coping with multiple demands and disruptions that resonated with what they say about the strained conditions of their work. While these complaints are of the mundane variety, there were indications of troubles that are far more deep-seated. Looking further leads us to conclude that hospitals are being restructured to accomplish goals that are not traditionally those of nurses, and the standpoint of nurses in the activities of caring is being subordinated. When nurses' work is organized outside of the everyday/everynight actualities, nurses are not free to act on their judgement. This may organize a more efficient hospital, but it reduces the value to be realized from employing a competent nursing staff.

It also results in a troubled nursing workforce. Nurses are responding in various ways within the limited options open to them. The steady rise of nurses' union activities and organized labour disruption are signs of the plight facing contemporary nursing (Sibbald 1999). At the end of a period of severe cutbacks in nursing, the turn of the century saw a serious shortage of nurses developing. Nurses were leaving the publicly funded system and moving their services into the private sector, both here in Canada and more so in the United States. Nurses have always moved about, and some have left nursing, looking for greener pastures, but in the early 2000s recruitment of new nurses also became challenging.[3] Rumblings of public opinion, caught recently on radio phone-in shows, indicate that the profession may no longer command the public trust and respect it enjoyed in earlier eras. Nurses have become a target for blame in explanations about 'what is wrong' with Canadian health care (Beardwood et al. 1999). People treat nurses' salary hikes and their more militant stance as self-serving and as evidence that nurses lack compassion and commitment. In the present public climate of scarcity, nurses' complaints about the conditions of their work and its financial remuneration are considered unseemly and socially unacceptable. One of our aims in this book is to help nurses reclaim the validity of their judgement – about their practice and what is happening to it.

When nurses are unhappy and frustrated they, too, blame others (whether front-line managers, middle managers, hospital executive staff, nursing teachers, government bureaucrats and politicians, or burned-out old nurses, as well as inexperienced new ones) for their current workplace and professional troubles. Nurses may conclude that hospital administrators do not understand the issues, plan poorly, make poor decisions, drain valuable resources away from direct practice, do not value or respect workers in direct care, and are ultimately responsible for the daily and nightly troubles of nurses. We have noticed that it is generally the case that problems with nurses, or problems raised by nurses, are construed by everybody involved to be issues of individual competency, commitment, and interpersonal relations. Organizational responses are made in this same mode. A recent trend in the new public management focuses on 'interpersonal conflict' (Gervase 2001; Annis Hammond 1998; Short 1998; Weisinger 1998). Thus framed, nurses' truculence is dealt with through programs developed to encourage leadership skills, foster effective communication skills, and to build 'effective teams.' These strategies are directed towards managing nurses' *expression* of their frustrations and worries. Typical of these strategies is the conflict management program that one regional health authority in British Columbia has instituted for dealing with such troubles. It seems that the notion of conflict can be used to identify any type of frustration that nurses (and their managers) express about their work. This includes the occasions when nurses are overwhelmed by the demands of their patients and the demands of the organization – or when nurses' new knowledge about discharges and bed utilization has not yet aligned them completely with the newly mandated practices of efficiency. We have noted many such circumstances that are disquieting to conscientious nurses. At the end of the day, they are likely to blame themselves. Nurses may have no way of resisting the designation of 'conflict,' since they feel conflicted and act on those feelings.

Telling the Truth

We are not persuaded by the accounts that blame individuals, nor by the remedies to which they lead. Our analytic goal has been to discover what is actually happening where nurses work and to ascertain how these settings have been organized (that way). Using institutional ethnography, we have the capacity to dissect the social organization of ordinary events through a research process of explication of the everyday world. Because it doesn't import and interpose theory between the ethnographic data and the account being offered, we say that we are 'telling the truth' (Smith 1999) about research settings. What is true and trustworthy within such research practices refers to the tracing and marshalling of material evidence to support an analytic account of the ethnographic data. It requires the researcher to follow an empirical process of discovery.

In this regard, we contrast our account of what is happening to the predominant characterization of what is going on (a characterization that appeared in our ethnographic data) that leads organizations to take up nurses' complaints as issues of 'a toxic climate' and then to manage 'conflict' and to 'change nurses' perceptions' of problems. That organizational approach frames what is going on in such a manner as to actually prevent nurses (and managers) from understanding and acting on the specific organizational circumstances of their troubles. We have come to the conclusion that until the untoward effects of administrative reforms are chronicled and legitimated by research that illuminates their socially organized character, nurses' responses will continue to be addressed as problems of individual incompetence, bad attitude, and poor communication. And nurses will continue to be expected to understand them that way. Our research contribution has been to show some of the actualities to which nurses are responding, as an alternative to focusing on and blaming them for feeling conflicted. Our method of knowing about nurses and Canadian health care 'tells the truth,' as we empirically track and carefully explicate the very ground of nurses' activities that shapes their work and their work lives.

To recapitulate what we have seen: perhaps most important is that the effects of restructuring are a significant component of the conflict that often grips nurses. Nurses themselves are being acted upon. They are being enrolled into the relations of ruling that are now being instituted in health care. Both nurses' knowing and acting are reconstituted thereby. Their subjectivity is being restructured as they activate the text-based and ideological practices of health care reform and hospital restructuring. We consider it important that nurses and others recognize that in activating the working texts, they absorb ruling ideas. Their place within the ruling agenda is crucial. Theirs is a bridging and coordinating position within the new order.

It is potentially devastating to the practice of nursing that nurses are so central to health care's new accounting logic. To make this argument, we have explicated the social organization of restructuring that hooks nurses into those textual practices, sometimes undermining nurses' capacity to enact the patient care that they judge to be required. We have described some ways that this happens, as nurses work with patient classification systems, quality assurance forms, bed-maps, alternate level of care texts, clinical pathways, and discharge planning flow sheets. In the absence of careful and critical analysis, these management technologies may appear to be specific to local conditions and needs, neutral tools that simply help nurses get their work done more efficiently and effectively. By tracking and analysing the texts that nurses activate, we were able to show how these (and we argue by logical extension, many other practices like them) engage nurses as subjects in strategies of reform. We made the argument that the discourse of efficiency, as constituted in managerial texts and in authorized organizational action, eventually overwhelms nurses' knowledge of patients as whole people. We were curious about how nurses learn to practice knowledgably this form of engagement that asks them to suspend their own professionally inculcated beliefs. We saw that they learn by doing. To engage in socially organized contemporary hospital settings, nurses must begin to see their patients in the hyper-real manner of the information technologies that constitute them as *objects* of managerial and professional action, including nurses' own action. As nurses participate in building and using this objectified knowledge of their patients, those very activities come to dominate their subsequent thinking and action. Some, and perhaps all nurses, will eventually learn to think this way, to *unconsciously* take for granted that objectified knowledge should supersede their own judgement. This is definitely the message they are being given. It advances the mode of knowing that dominates health care today.

Yet, at every turn, we meet contradictions within health care restructuring. Consider this. The technologies that reorganize patient care are meant to be understood as part of an effort to sustain the public provision of health care in Canada. As instituted within the accounting logic of new public management strategies, health care is expected to be managed more precisely, using the new knowledge capacity not only for more efficient, timely, and effective use of resources – but for greater accountability. A huge investment in information technologies is intended to provide an accurate and objective basis for making all sorts of decisions for governance, management, and therapeutics. This mind-boggling array of new text-based technologies and the reforms they guide would seem to be directed towards the 'public good' – the provision of good, accessible, sustainable health care. Many studies reflect their apparent successes.[4] Into this discourse, we insert a different perspective, in which we highlight what we see as inherent dangers. Our analysis draws attention to instances of the approach to knowing objectively that is at the heart of the new public management, infusing the health care system with its own meanings. We want people to recognize that the new public management should be thought of as a complex ruling apparatus that draws nurses into its web of ruling practices and purposes. We see in this the capacity of a ruling agenda to reconfigure and erode, not just nursing, but 'the public good,' at least as we have known it in Canada.

It is important that our critique not be misunderstood. It would be too easy to dismiss our analysis for what it does not say about the wide-ranging benefits of new technologies. We value, as hospital and nurse managers do, efficiency in work and in the use of resources, effective treatments, equity and timeliness of access to care, and the dedication of health care practitioners to patients and to their quality of care. We count on having access to such care for ourselves and our friends and families when necessary, now and in the future. Our concern is that the increasing, and almost exclusive, reliance on information-based technologies for making decisions in hospitals produces a knowledge disjuncture between those who have the authorized 'facts' and those whose lives are being regulated by them. Certain facts are authorized; others are subjugated. And – here is the rub – being socially organized, facts can be marshalled for partisan purposes. Green (2004) sees the potential for conflict of interest as administrative staff prepare reports to inform a regional health board whose responsibility it is to evaluate their performance; she points out that choices are made by administrators about what to include in the reports and what 'to make of' those data. We have argued in a similar vein that when the managerial need for knowledge establishes the conceptual framing of what is known, the account constructed bears that imprint. This has many potential and actual consequences.

We also noted that the social organization of health information is not, as Timmermans and Berg seem to argue, an issue that can be remedied by scrutinizing more closely *how* the technologies should be put to work in order to more fully account for and address the 'different universalities' (2003: 200) encountered across health care settings. Scrupulous consideration is already being given to how the technologies are implemented locally and how 'different universalities' are recognized. We observed, in the different hospitals and health regions we studied, each clinical pathway, discharge planning protocol, ALC designation process, or patient classification system being rethought in relation to its deployment, with careful attention being given to local contexts and input from the individual professionals affected. Yet, as Mykhalovskiy and Weir (2004) argue, efforts such as these leave aside any interrogation of the 'knowledge mechanics' at work. In the sort of knowing used to produce protocols to standardize a worksite, any knowledge disjuncture organized and any power relation embedded are left unexamined. Maintaining the current belief in and dependence on the established, scientized, and nominalized forms of information and organization (despite the implementation modifications proposed by Timmermans and Berg) perpetuates the disjunctures about which we are concerned.

We have been especially interested in the more or less unassailable status of the information generated within various organizational technologies. We have analysed some of the information generated and have made empirically based arguments against the assumption that it always supplies the best basis for action (that is, for people as opposed to an organizational agenda) in health care settings. We propose that there is much to learn from *what is actually happening* in the activities of the people 'on the ground' of health care. We have argued that what people know experientially needs to be legitimated instead of repudiated, that the pendulum has swung too far in the so-called scientific direction (that is, the scientifically authorized, objectified, direction). In this regard, the claim to a scientific basis for any knowledge about health care generates the requirement that it be evaluated as science is, and that is what we are beginning to do.

We have illuminated how virtual accounts dominate actual settings – that's the appeal of the approach within the new public management. It remakes local settings in the image of the virtual account with, we have argued, both good and bad effects. We have insisted that readers understand how the pressures to achieve standardized efficiencies compete with the individual needs of patients as nurses might know them. We have warned that the deleterious effects of these new practices are not usually available for examination or action within established knowledge practices of the new public management. In that regard, we have exposed the circularity of knowing that organizes what is happening in clinical settings in coherence with virtual accounts that carry pre-established schemata of efficiency and quality. This is the outstanding and, from some perspectives, the 'successful' feature of the technologies that we describe. In these systems, the production of facts – that which can be known legitimately – can *only* be framed from within the established schemata. The practical activities of health care can be regulated thereby, with the textual hyper-reality standing in for what is actually happening – at least for organizational purposes. Whatever else is going on is rendered invisible, not legitimately knowable nor actionable.

A long-standing concern for nurses has been the invisibility of, and lack of recognition accorded to, much of their work.[5] They carry on with the work anyway, guided by nursing scholarship, personal commitments, and professional expectations. Their experiences of working from such aspirations, beliefs, and knowledge constitute nursing judgement and convey what we speak of as the standpoint of caring.

But, through conducting the research reported here, we have come to recognize that nurses' consciousness is being reorganized away from their traditional standpoint in the expression of caring. The domination of the ruling practices accomplishes this. Socialized and trained to care for people, nurses are now being taught, coached, and persuaded that it is their professional duty to nurse the organization.

We have been impressed by some ways in which we saw this happening. Nursing within organizational priorities could be said to be professionally sanctioned by, among other things, use of particular language such as our examples of the use of the concept of holism, transposed from nursing to organizational texts. In the blending of what we called speech genres, new authoritative uses of language sidetrack nurses' attention and shift their beliefs. This blended language use provides the discursive terrain in which nurses can 'speak good nursing' while practising something else. In the texts we analysed we noted references such as 'efficiency in caring,' 'accountability,' and 'responsibility' being used in a double-sided way. They evoked nurses' *own* (altruistic) professional ideas while reinforcing nurses' conception that controlling costs, emptying beds, and rationing their caring attention are legitimate nursing interests of the highest priority. Nurses are expected, both as caring nurses and as caring citizens, to respond to the need for cost reductions in order to achieve the ' best advantages for patients and society' (Sandhu, Duquette, and Kérouac 1992: 34). Our appraisal of several professional nursing texts produced exhibits of nurses' language constructing a kind of idealized image of the profession, the work, and nurses' commitments, to which nurses, reading it, would expect themselves to conform; we noticed that, at the same time, the language imperceptibly builds in and justifies nurses' complicity with a ruling standpoint.

We have begun to uncover how within the new public management 'the public' is an endangered terrain. Others share our concern about this. Zygmunt Bauman (2003, paraphrased by Jelly-Shapiro 2004: 73) cautions that in a world governed by neoliberal capitalism, the sense of a 'public' is disappearing, replaced by the vulgarities of private interests. Bauman's argument is that people are made surplus when privatization and the production of efficiencies streamline the economic activities of the day; the technologies of efficiency produce surplus populations who exist at the margins of the systems of consumption. One immediately thinks about downsizing and contracting out of jobs that reduce the employed health labour force, throwing experienced and dedicated workers into underemployment or unemployment. But there is another way to see how the restructuring of health services creates surplus populations. 'As the public becomes privatized, the lives of the excess are no longer noticed; they, with all their particularities, disappear' (Bauman, cited by Jelly-Shapiro 2004: 74). Our own analysis builds an account of the particularities of patients who are marginalized when efficiency measures constitute them in terms of their cost-relevant parts. As whole bodies and as subjectivities, they become excess. All that is needed to work on them is knowledge of them as parts, as objects, expressed commensurably. Patients' individualized needs, their experiences of symptoms, and their human suffering are relegated to the 'surplus.' Strategies are put into place to standardize and streamline and manage efficiently these sorts of 'surplus.' Yet, throughout the decades of reform and restructuring, patients have looked to nurses to treat them as whole people who continue to experience pain and hope, breathlessness, nausea, and fever. They continue to need attention to their suffering, their feelings of vulnerability, and their experiences of fear. The sort of work that nurses would have done to address patients' (now excess) needs is being squeezed out. Or it is relegated to a volunteer, or to an instruction sheet, or often to a family member, if a patient is lucky enough to have one close by. As nurses and their work are brought within this erosion of the public good, we understand it creates a serious contradiction for them – and their patients.

Not just nurses but members of the public, too, are being incorporated into the thinking about health care within the framework of the new public management. As we write, 'accessibility' and 'waiting' are being turned into topics of interest for mass media consumption. Provincial and territorial recipients of new federal funding are required to report 'to their residents on health system performance' (HCA 2004 website).[6] Issues of performance and, in this case, accessibility, no doubt have resonance for many Canadians who are themselves or have family and friends waiting for joint replacements, MRIs, angioplasties, or consultations with medical specialists. The question we think it important to keep our eye on is 'How does the new public management approach to 'waiting' sweep us further into the restructuring of care that satisfies interests other than our own?' It is going to be difficult to determine this when what we can know, for instance, about 'wait-times,' is already worked up within forms of knowledge intrinsic to a ruling project.

Here is one example of that problem. In British Columbia the public has been given access to 'waiting list' data posted on the Ministry of Health website. As well, a recent provincial survey of emergency departments included 'waiting times' as part of how respondents were to rate emergency care. And premiers' conferences have highlighted and compared 'waiting times' across the provincial boundaries. All these events make 'news' of various statistics about waiting for health care. In British Columbia this attention to waiting list statistics supports a strategy whereby the use of private hospital facilities becomes the solution to the problems that hospitals may have in managing their waiting lists. In 2004–5, in British Columbia, 1,000 surgeries were being contracted out to private facilities.[7] 'Not waiting' has become a legitimate and even lauded justification for public payment of private health care provision. That is, information on waiting times is readily absorbed into a rationale, amplified by the media, for eroding the public health care system. All this adds weight to our view that socially organized knowledge (reports, data sets, and such) that give concepts such as 'waiting' their particular features requires careful mapping in order to tell the truth about what is happening.

People expect that more accountability will strengthen health care and improve its administration. We too strongly favour more transparency in how health care funds are used. Our scepticism comes in when we look at the success of performance reporting as accountability; it arises from the built-in flaw in methods that rely on the managerial work-up of the facts within information systems that blend cost and quality accounting. Intrinsic to accountability practices is the socially organized knowledge that they operate upon. 'Knowing' is never neutral, and health system datasets are constructed from managerial information that is already formed to fit existing interpretive and processing frameworks. Managerial accountability practices, formulating knowledge of health care within an orientation to measure and control it, offer a different view from what might be learned if knowing were to begin, for instance, from nurses' everyday/everynight location. As can be extrapolated from our analysis of a patient satisfaction survey, systematic technologies relied upon to gauge accountability will also construct a particular picture of what is actually happening in health care. Any such accountability process will rely on managerial information that is distanced and insulated from the peopled settings – where people fall ill, suffer accidents, recover, or succumb. Its conceptualization, like that of other objectified information about patients, is within the ruling framework. Constructed as virtual reality, such accountability will not express what is happening *on the ground* of health care.

Where This Leads – Alternative Accounts and Oppositional Work

Our mapping of the relations that organize the everyday/everynight actualities of hospital care identifies the ruling relations of health information. We have emphasized the organizing capacities of information within restructuring. We have signalled how health information is central to the new public management in building a new kind of organization for the provision of health care. And, in that regard, we have made critical arguments about the unquestioning belief in and use of objective information. Our analysis of what is happening shows people working in competitively organized health care settings, bringing their activities into line with new ideas about managing care. The forms of knowledge that coordinate their activities are to some extent (still) in contention, still being innovated. But at the same time, we showed the systematic manner in which certain objectified knowledge triumphs over knowledge arising from embodied practice. The ethnographic attention we brought to bear on nurses at work shows that their proximity to actual patients informs their practice differently, troubling their conversion into the new work practices that are guided textually and, apparently, objectively. Yet, there is an imbalance in the power associated with different accounts. Our argument is not that we should return to some apparently golden age when health care authorities might rely on doctors' and nurses' expertise exclusively, as in some earlier forms of professional control of health care. That had and would still have its own problems. For instance, the nurses we observed are also being changed, their consciousness reorganized, their knowing restructured. As professionals and professional regulators are being absorbed into the ruling relations and the various spheres of activity blended, nurses' knowing comes to reflect that emerging state of affairs.

This complicates what we can say about knowing, about what can be known and relied on, within the new health care regime. Our analysis directs us to treat experiential knowing as the key to what is missing. That is not to say that nurses' 'hands on' knowledge can compete successfully with managerial knowledge for use within the contemporary structures of health care management and governance. The institution in which nursing happens generates the particular knowledge that guides its activities, and today's nurses are not separate and cannot separate themselves from those virtual accounts. They connect the local settings into the broad web of Canadian health information and into funding and accountability structures. Nurses' own practical knowledge won't work in the same way as text-mediated accounts, and thus it won't be valued in the same way. This is not a matter of individual choice, nor of options that can be exercised by individual administrators who are sensitive to nurses. It also flies in the face of efforts within several of the hospitals that we studied, where 'nursing practice councils' and 'nursing advisory boards' include representatives from nurses in direct practice. Were we to assume the opposite, that nurses' experiential knowing would be accepted and treated as equal to and of the same relevance as objectified information, we might argue for an accommodation of the standpoint of nurses' knowledge within the decision-making practices of hospital administration, for a reconciliation between the different ways of knowing. Of course, professionals have expertise that health care organizations need and do use. However, merely including nurses in the decision-making structure of administration does not counteract how their managers and hospital administrators, and increasingly nurses, too, are agents of the ruling relations of health care. The reform agenda and its restructuring strategies (clinical pathways, patient satisfaction surveys, growing ambulatory care programs, bed closures, and so forth) will operate, as we have shown them to do, no matter what nurses' advisory councils advise. As the objectified form of health care knowledge generated in coherence with objective management becomes increasingly dominant, *the practices it supports rule out traditional ways of knowing and acting*. Knowledges are valued differently precisely because of their different utility for managing objectively. The question remains, when knowledges clash, can they be used simultaneously? Can they be harmonized?

Our findings suggest that, at least for nurses, the answer is no. The activities that we describe throughout this book chronicle almost thirty years of the unfolding events of hospital restructuring. Much of what has been accomplished during this time seems irrevocably entrenched – a tide impossible to turn back. Nurses' consciousness has been altered, ideas about efficiency are firmly ingrained, nurses' professional regulatory bodies are generating and using their own brand of abstracted, information-based technologies to regulate and monitor nursing practices. While nurses' empirical knowledge is still used alongside other, objective ways of knowing, we have argued that the latter disorganizes and colonizes the former. Our sense is that in such an environment, oppositional work supportive of patient care is called for.

What our analysis makes possible is a way to 'talk back' (Smith 1987) to forms of knowledge that misrepresent the everyday/everynight world and undermine patient care. This direction highlights the practical usefulness of *alternative* accounts. Our analytic work on the social relations of nurses' work within the new public management makes a beginning. Mapping the empirical ground on which nursing is done contrasts with the knowledge for management that works up those actualities into virtual accounts. Note that our map also contrasts with and goes beyond 'what nurses know' from their everyday/everynight involvement in the workplace. Our analysis puts in place an alternative from which to consider first, *how* things are being organized and then, in the situations we explored, how that social organization works against nurses and against patients. We have already said that alternative accounts do not replace knowledge for management. Nor do they replace nurses' professional education, the knowledge base of their professional judgement. But, as a first and important step, alternative accounts such as ours do legitimize nurses' experience as a basis for reading and interpreting their organized work settings from nurses' standpoint.

Learning about experience as an authoritative basis of knowing suggests how to take action on particular issues, and it has important implications for nurse educators. It can tie nurses' knowing about what actually happens to how these things get taken up, transformed, and returned to the workplace in information that dominates nursing. This is a form of knowing that can help nursing instructors reflect on the way nursing education plays a part in ruling relations, in creating new participants who are willing and able to contribute to the ruling project(s). Indeed, without an alternative account, new nurses may be altruistic but completely unprepared to resist being absorbed by ruling ideas. Education is an important site of opposition to the erosion of nurses' judgement; and it is important to remember that even under contemporary methods of management, hospitals are still substantially reliant on nurses' judgement. This is the stage upon which nurses' oppositional work can be performed on behalf of their patients. Nurses write their patients into organizational accounts – always a judgement and a knowledge-based decision. But the moulding of students towards compliance with ruling practices begins early in their student careers. They are trained to recognize as nursing, and appreciate as theirs, the responsibility to concert their actions with the relevancies being inserted into nursing through the new public management. Campbell describes how nurses are taught accountability practices in their nursing education. Her research of an instructional program empirically traced how nursing students learn 'to be adequate account-makers,' that is, how they are taught to scan their experiences at work in order 'to cover all the documentary bases, *creating the appearance* of adequate nursing action' (1995: 232, emphasis in original). This appears to be preparing them to conceptualize nursing for professional interpretation and recording purposes. What is less apparent is that it is also the training that allows them to play their necessary part in transposing nursing actualities into the managerial information that reorganizes their work (Campbell and Jackson 1992). Nurse educators persuaded by our analysis are well positioned to develop curricula to offer students analytic skills to question, 'Whose knowledge are we authorizing?' 'In whose interests does this knowledge work?' 'What knowledge does it displace?'

An illustration of this point comes from Janet Rankin and Linda Shorting, a nursing colleague, who are currently developing a course that will introduce second- and third-year nursing students to the authorized work of discharge planning. The students will learn the roles and responsibilities of discharge planning nurses as they liaise with families and community agencies. The student practicum will focus on the nursing care of patients who are being prepared for discharge. The students' practice is intended to offer them opportunities to develop relationships with patients and also to consolidate their learning about physical assessment, pathophysiology, diagnostic tests, pharmacology, and so forth (important components of the second- and third-year nursing curricula). But the students' practice will also develop a critical analysis of how discharge planning and its intersections with family, community supports, and so forth, may disrupt what the student had understood should be done. Guided critical reflection offers students an alternative account of the (otherwise taken for granted) organizational order, and it generates the legitimacy for them to reconceptualize and query it.

Analysing instructional work in the academy should make nursing faculty members acutely aware of how an education in the human service professions provides students with the conceptual tools to *rationalize* their participation in the ruling relations of professional work. Nursing curricula now offer conceptual tools that allow students to leap (conceptually) to producing 'proper' written accounts of their experiences. Yet, instead of being rewarded for adopting and moving seamlessly into the textual environment of nursing's objective management, students could be taught how to separate out the different interests appearing in the work. They could learn to recognize as moments for their knowledgeable intervention the mismatches between what happens and the accounts they are to make of it. Such disjunctures, which in their classrooms can be treated as abstract issues, do not disappear when students are working on wards. They rise up and trouble students. Nursing students, like the graduates they will become, have to handle them as best they can and accept the consequences.

Instructive, in this regard, is one student's experience of caring for an eighteen-year-old woman who had just given birth to her second child. After a particularly difficult labour, the weary patient refused to have her infant sleep beside her. She also complained that the other moms and babes sharing her four-bed room kept her awake. Sympathizing with her restlessness, the student decided to 'sneak' this new mother (almost a child herself) into an empty private room for the night. The staff and the supervising instructor were critical of this intervention, explaining how it did not fit the new philosophy of maternal-child care (geared towards the promotion of breastfeeding that includes, in most hospitals, the closure of well-baby nurseries). Moreover, the student was told, it was not a fair distribution of hospital resources because it could not be offered to all the other mothers who could not afford to pay for a private room. One nurse also explained that despite the fact that the patient slept in her own bed in the private room, the intervention breached principles of asepsis because it would not be possible to get a housekeeper to clean the bathroom for the next patient to be admitted. The student's apparently creative and individualized response to her patient's fatigue was conceptualized and criticized through interpretive frameworks that prioritized other interests. This is an instance of a student being coached to account for her practice within a rationalizing professional framework that she knew was not adequate to her caring concerns.

Lacking an alternative account, this nursing student was guided towards an uncaring response. If she and her mentors had had the knowledge basis for an alternative account they might have noticed when efficiency practices work against patients and nurses and how they have become taken for granted as authoritative. They might be able to reclaim their experience of how this chafes, as it produces a disjuncture between their caring commitments and the inexorable unfolding of so-called hospital efficiency. It is in this disjunctive space that an analysis for oppositional work can begin for nurses, within the terrain of their practical activity. It is here where possibilities for social action can be sparked – taking up the standpoint of nurses, in the interest of their patients. An alternative account insulates nurses, not against meeting text-based ruling in their workplaces, but against being overwhelmed intellectually by how these technologies are designed to dominate the local setting.

Alternative accounts do not come ready-to-hand, but must be researched and developed. There is much analysis waiting to be done. Ours offers just a beginning. The ground of health care changes all the time, and accounts, to remain true to that, have to be updated continually. Opportunities for such research exist within institutes, departments, and schools of sociology, politics, and policy studies, nursing and health studies, health information science, health sciences research, epidemiology, and others. Much of the funding for health care research assumes the implicit goodness of the methods for organizing health care provision that we criticize. Given its standpoint, the funding provides for research to elaborate, extend, and test the operation of such methods, rarely to analyse them critically. Even evaluation takes place within the interpretive framework that we criticize here. We have uncovered some of the hidden jeopardy that these prevailing knowledge-based approaches cannot reveal, as researchers work within their ruling and ideological frameworks.

Our perspective on this goes against the grain of a good deal of contemporary belief, not just in health care and public management, but as explained in the Introduction to this book, in research practice. We accept that any criticism of current information and management or governance technologies and the practices they support must be substantiated on the basis of evidence. Our evidence is of a different sort from that supplied through randomized controlled trials. But it is evidence nonetheless. We look at and bring readers with us, through our ethnographic descriptions, into the various settings where people actually interact, where programs are put in place, where health care actually happens. On this empirical basis, we draw attention to what works and what doesn't, what is being lost from, and what is being added to the ruling accounts, generated as they are with identifiable conceptual structures already given, matching ruling purposes and principles. Our analysis makes explicit the connections that otherwise never appear.

This explicative approach must be applied not just to work settings and their social organization, but to the specially constructed information that is integral to the operation and maintenance of those settings and the provision of care within them. As our analysis shows, health information is an artefact that, among its other important characteristics, includes its 'facticity.' Herein lies a major concern for all those who are persuaded by our social organization of knowledge argument. Currently health information is accepted as representing accurately to decision-makers what happens in practice. In constructing health information, there are requirements of adequate methodology to be followed, but we insist that they are not sufficient to guarantee its trustworthiness. As we have argued throughout this book, the following issue is still left unattended: 'Any questions bearing on the facticity of statements based on the intersection of data and interpretive schema (such as issues of accuracy, reliability, and the like) may be raised without breaking the ideological circularity of the procedure. ... Issues, questions and experiences that do not fit the framework ... simply do not get entry to the process, do not become part of the textual realities governing the decision-making processes' (Smith 1990a: 93–4).

This observation should be unsettling to the hopes of federal bureaucrats and health care advocates for whom 'reporting' to the Canadian people stands as the sine qua non of accountability, for example, how accountability has been explicitly outlined in directions for the deployment of recent federal health grants (CHA 2004). We have also cited Green's (2004) research that suggests how data categories and indicators may be selected to build a particular picture, perhaps one that reflects positively on those who are responsible for the entity being reported. We have offered instances of other routine construction flaws hidden in so-called objective data and the reports that they inform. This is an area that desperately needs further research attention. To overlook the difficulties that arise when virtual realities lift away from the actualities of the everyday life that they purport to represent is to court disaster in health care. We propose ethnographically informed explication (or perhaps, deconstruction) of the social organization of the information that is increasingly treated as the product of the Canadian health care system. Accountability focusing on such textual products may accomplish its ruling purposes but otherwise fail people and, moreover, obscure that failure.

How we know determines what we can see. More importantly, it determines what we can see to be a problem. For researchers, our work is to continue to 'join the dots' and advance an analysis of how the new public management is working. None of us can accomplish this work in isolation. Unless we do take up this challenge, it will become increasingly difficult to protect the values embedded in the Canadian health care system. Already the traditional value that Canadians have always placed on collective responsibility is under serious challenge. Various kinds of 'mass think' and demagoguery chip away at what we believe is possible and right. In this regard, developing the capacity to analyse how things work can be seen to be a contribution to the health of our democracy. The same applies for learning how knowledge works. Information is a social product and how it does or does not conform to what it purports to represent can and must be examined. The critically important asset available to those who work in the health care system, as nurses do, is that they are on the ground where things actually happen. Experiential knowing is an irreplaceable resource for the ethnographic analysis of information that we are recommending be conducted. When all of us can make sense of our experience, we don't have to rely solely on what experts (or the media) tell us. That may help us in efforts to hold on to our public health care system.

This book has mapped some of the new features appearing in nurses' work lives over the past few decades. If in the course of this analysis we seem to be celebrating nurses and nursing, that is a reading with which we are content. We recognize and have wanted to emphasize the responsibility that nurses carry. At the same time, we have argued that nursing is being transformed and new contradictions are entering nursing work, altering nurses' standpoint. The standpoint of nurses, which we have also called the standpoint of caring, insofar as it expresses care for the people nurses meet as patients, is organized by the relations within which nursing happens. The analysis shows that nurses must do their work within the specific relations of health care that they enter as its participants. Those relations shift and change all the time, carrying nurses with them. What caring becomes is also socially organized in this manner. This creates not just a problem for nursing and individual nurses, but also a new kind of responsibility. Being there, where health care policy and funding are translated into action, being not just a caregiver but a witness, is both a privilege and an opportunity. To take up that opportunity nurses need to understand about being an insider in an institution and a profession that is being restructured by new ruling relations. Our contribution in this book is to help nurses recognize their unusual positioning – both *in* the ruling relations and yet held to the actualities of their patients' lives by being there with them. Because nurses' positioning is never absolute and fixed with regard to enacting a caring versus a ruling standpoint, theirs is a unique and dynamic location. Their experiential knowing offers nurses the capacity to know health care and speak about it from a standpoint organized differently from that of those who rule it. On this basis we want to encourage nurses to make their voices heard about what they know to be happening in Canada's health care system.

Notes

Introduction

1 The 'theory-practice gap' is the current formulation of the problem (Gallagher 2004; Harris 2004). In the 1970s and 1980s it was talked about as 'reality shock' (Kramer 1974; 1981).

2 Burn-out is described as a 'psychological state resulting from ineffective strategies for coping with and enduring stress' (Ekstedt and Fagerberg 2005: 59).

3 Readers trained in the information disciplines will notice that we do not follow their conventions of language use (specifically, the definitions of 'knowledge,' 'information,' and 'data'). Nurses, too, accept these definitions; see, e.g., Curran and Gassert who quote Blum (1986: 35): '*Data* are discrete entities that describe objectively without interpretation. *Information* is data that are interpreted, organized, or structured. *Knowledge* is synthesized information in which interrelationships are identified and formalized' (1998: 65; emphasis in original). This is in contrast to our own analytic attempts to discover how these words mean different things to different people depending on their social settings of use.

4 Models of nursing (e.g., Henderson 1966; King 1981; Orem 1979; Roy and Roberts 1981) on which curricula were based in the 1960s to 1980s have been replaced by increasingly sophisticated conceptualizations of nurse-and-patient interactions. Nurses are now being taught to take into account the dynamics and emergent nature of patients' experiences as central to nursing decisionmaking (Petri 2005; Haylor 2000), and this coalesces in curricula with evidence-based practice models.

5 We are using this term to point to the specific and organized efforts to manage organizations 'professionally.' By this we mean employing management

professionals, not management *of* professional health care practitioners *by* professionals from within similar disciplines. Indeed, the changes in health care organizations that managerialism accomplishes 'reflect a distrust of professional autonomy' (Broadbent and Laughlin 2002: 101).

6 Such as Margaret Thatcher's acclaimed and widely copied 'resolve to reshape a sluggish British economy and a lethargic public sector' (Borins 2002: 182).

7 'Accounting logic' is built on two assumptions: (1) that any activity needs to be evaluated in terms of some measurable outputs achieved and the value added in the course of any activity; and (2) that it is possible to undertake this evaluation in and through the financial resources actually used or received (Broadbent and Laughlin 2002: 101).

8 Reading institutional ethnography without a background in this approach to doing social analysis can be made more difficult than it should be by our (writers') use of technical language. As in any other research approach, technical language is not simply decorative, but plays an integral part in how the analysis is done and how it must be described. We have tried to reduce to just the essentials our specialized language use and to use those words in a context that, by and large, we think is self-explanatory. However, that is not to say that all is explained in the chapters of this book. We are particularly aware that institutional ethnography calls on those who do it, and also on those who read it, to look at the world in a certain way. Let's say, to begin, that we bring to our research certain assumptions both about the world and about what is interesting to learn about it from research. So, although any institutional ethnography starts with the consideration of data collected by ordinary ethnographic methods (observations and interviews, for instance), it uses those data for analytic purposes that display how (those and other related instances of) everyday life are organized. To elaborate: along with analysts of many other persuasions, institutional ethnographers believe that the social world is socially organized; that people bring the social into being. It is in people's work that we can see the 'social relations' that institutional ethnographers talk about. Given that we understand social life to be constituted through 'people acting,' the focus of our analysis must be on what actual people actually do. But our interest in them and their doings is not simply in studying discrete settings or sequences of action, but rather in how their local activity is hooked into larger processes that, in turn, make up the society that we live in. Or we can turn that around: institutional ethnographers want to be able to discover how social relations arising elsewhere organize the local doings of our informants. This brings us to the major theoretical assumption of institu-

tional ethnography, that is, that social life, in this postindustrial, capitalist, and globally organized society is organized by ruling relations; when people are constituting their everyday lives, they do so knowledgeably, in concert with and in ways dictated by ruling relations. This belief leads to the specific kind of research or analytic interest that motivates institutional ethnography. Institutional ethnographers attempt to find out *how things work*. They do not speculate on the causes of things and design research projects to test hypotheses. Rather, they focus analytic attention, empirically, on the material world – of people doing things, making things happen, of actual lives lived in actual settings. This is how the concept of 'standpoint' is used by institutional ethnographers; it is the point where *those* real people 'stand,' and the location from which *those* people's knowledge and activities (in this case the knowledgeable activities of nurses in direct practice) are organized. The big question in institutional ethnography is always about how everyday/everynight life there, in that setting, is organized to happen as it does. To get such answers, means moving beyond the experiential accounts that informants in *that* setting may provide. Institutional ethnographers follow the clues they uncover 'on the ground' as they lead (connect) into the 'outside world.' This interest directs other kinds of data collection. Using clues from the ethnographic data, the researcher now looks at 'the institutional.' She looks for evidence of how ruling practices are organizing the local setting; she must learn about ruling apparatuses and discourses and the knowledgeable activities of those who administer and operate them. And it is in following this interest that texts become so important to institutional ethnographers. Texts are ubiquitous features of our kind of society, and we all are involved in activating them – putting ourselves into the textual accounts we encounter. We know how to use such texts or we learn how, because we must – in order to perform our everyday lives adequately. As we do, besides operating the (textual) technologies of institutional life through which we access the benefits of health care, the legal system, employment and compensation, holding property, etc., we also are regulated by those same and other textual practices. We engage with texts knowledgeably and absorb and perform the coordination that they carry into our lives and activities. We read our mail, including our Visa bills, and monthly we pay our debts, manipulating paper and computer texts competently. We pick a piece of paper off our car's windscreen and engage with the justice system, paying our parking fines, and on time, too, or we suffer the consequences. Such examples identify ruling practices that are commonplace. They also identify the competencies with which we operate in the text-mediated world. But much of what happens to us just seems to happen. Its complexity is not available to be seen and understood. How it happens, how it has been organized to catch us up in ruling practices that guide our actions, even guide our knowing and our explanations of our actions, is and remains mysterious. Such social organization may remain unquestioned until a specialized form of analysis makes the connections between our experience and how it happens. This is the kind of discovery that institutional ethnography has been developed to make possible. Dorothy E. Smith's *The Everyday World as Problematic* (1987), *Institutional Ethnography: A Sociology for People* (2005), and Marie Campbell's and Frances Gregor's *Mapping Social Relations: A Primer in Doing Institutional Ethnography* (2002) offer more detailed help.

9 Health care analyst Michael Rachlis praises managerial innovation highly, claiming that only innovation will save public health care. Osborne and Plastrik place 'innovation' within the strategies of the new public management and entrepreneurial government that they explain as 'the fundamental transformation of public systems and organizations to create dramatic increases in their effectiveness, efficiency, adaptability, and capacity to innovate, [such] transformation [being[accomplished by changing their purpose, accountability, incentives, power structure, and culture' (2000: 4).

10 But consider similarly critical analyses of other public programming, e.g., McCoy (1999), on public post-secondary education, or Jackson (2005), on publicly funded literacy programs.

11 See Janet M. Rankin's unpublished doctoral dissertation (2004) and articles published in 2001 and 2003.

12 See Marie L. Campbell's unpublished doctoral dissertation (1984) and other research by Campbell published in 1988, 1992, 1994, 1995, 1998, 2000, and 2001, for which Campbell gratefully acknowledges funding from National Health and Welfare Canada, Social Sciences and Humanities Research Council of Canada, Human Resource Development Canada, and the Juan de Fuca Hospital Society

1 The Managerial Turn in Nursing

1 Canada's National Medicare Program was inaugurated on 1 July 1968; provinces and territories joined the program over the next four years (Taylor 1978: 375).

2 The Hospital Insurance and Diagnostic Services Act, passed in 1957, and by 1961, 'ten provincial plans were melded into the reality of a national program' (Taylor 1978: 234).

3 The criteria to govern the operation of Medicare are usually listed as uni-

versality, comprehensiveness, equitability, portability, and public adminis-tration. See e.g., Fuller (1998: 73–4), for a discussion of what these loosely defined criteria mean for service provision.

4 Among many possible examples is the following: The Canadian Health Coalition notes critically how Senator Michael Kirby, an influential voice in health care reform, and at the same time a director of a private health care firm, acts for the Canadian people in political and judicial forums in spite of the apparent conflicts in these roles.

5 For example, British Columbia's was reported in 1993, Nova Scotia's in 1989, and Ontario's in 1991.

6 But such talk has a highly political and polemic character. For a different view, see Carol Goar's article, 'Doctor's Orders: Grain of Salt,' in the *Toronto Star*, 13 Aug. 2004.

7 *Links*, the newsletter of the Canadian Health Services Research Foundation (CHSRF) states in its Mythbusters section (Spring 2001), that 'wildly differ-ent claims for waiting times' can be explained by 'the capricious nature of waiting times data.'

8 Haynes et al. (1995) delineated one approach to making stronger, more workable, links between evidence and practice. In 2000, the CHSRF notes its commitment to 'linkage and exchange' between applied researchers and decision makers in health organizations (2000: 1) and it thereafter changed its newsletter's name to *Links* (from *Quid Novi*), said to 'reflect the founda-tion's central role.'

9 Established in 1997 with endowed funds from federal sources, the CHSRF is a national not-for-profit corporation whose mandate is to service the research needs of health system policymakers and managers. Its 1999 Annual Report states: 'There is every sign that the national debate on healthcare will intensify as provincial and federal governments continue to struggle over the future of the healthcare system. The need for sound evi-dence to guide that debate will therefore grow, and the kinds of programs the foundation supports have a crucial role in supplying that evidence' (1999a: 7).

10 Officially launched in June 2000, CIHR's expenditures for that budget year ending March 2001 were $370 million for research and $20 million for administration (CIHR 2000–1).

11 The CHSRF newsletter (1999b: 1) used this phrase in reporting on 'interest in indicators that measure performance' of many systems and services in health care and in commenting on the '$95 million over three years to the CIHI to develop more and improved indicators of the performance of Can-ada's health systems and the health of the population.'

12 In 1982, 64 of 165 Ontario hospitals responding to a survey (a 74 per cent response rate) were using patient classification systems in planning and forecasting, scheduling staff, and budgeting nursing hours; 42 more Ontario hospitals reported that they were in the planning phase of introducing patient classification (Ontario Hospital Association 1982).

13 This legislation reduced the federal government's transfer payments to provinces for health care from 50 per cent to an amount that varied in relation to GNP.

14 The closing of hospital nursing schools beginning in the 1960s, and the loss of their free or low-paid student labour pool increased the pressure for more rigorous methods of managing nursing staffing.

15 The account given in this chapter draws on doctoral research (Campbell 1984). One hospital's nursing information and management systems were studied as an entry point for analysing how a nursing labour process *could be influenced* through use of such information-based methods. More than a case study, the research offers an analysis of the managerial processes through which funding processes link specific policies to definite outcomes in geographically dispersed organizations. One particular patient classification system, from a possible dozen or so that were in common use across the country at the time, was analysed and described. The claim made for this study is that regardless of the particularities of these systems, the *processes* described are the same wherever this kind of information-based technology of management is used.

16 A popular version of the rationale by journalists Bennett and Krasny appeared in a series entitled 'Health-Care in Canada' in a Toronto newspaper (*Financial Post*, 26 March to 7 May 1977).

17 Accounting analysts such as Chua are sceptical that the numbers produced through managerial accounting systems actually relate very closely to the hospital activities and the patients that they claim to represent. Chua argues that the social manufacture of accounting data does, however, alter power relations, transferring dominance to those who can claim, on the basis of the data, to 'know' more (1991: 31). This is the crux of the argument being presented here in relation to nurses: the new knowledge of patients' needs for nursing care that patient classification generates alter the structure of decisionmaking about nurse staffing. Beyond that, as developed in this analysis, are the personal costs to nurses and patients that such a transformation of effort, power, and control introduces.

18 Jackson (2005), uses this term when describing how literacy workers deal with new public management expectations. Continued funding may depend upon them accounting for aspects of their work in numerical

'results' – even when workers know such results to be both non-quantifi-
able and unachievable in the time-frames in question. This is when literacy
workers are likely to 'game' the results.

19 In early versions of the patient classification form, and before the system's
computerization, a cardboard template was applied to each filled-out form
to reveal the classification numbers.

20 The patient classification systems attempt to respond to these exigencies by
the addition of a definite amount of time said to be for 'indirect' nursing
care. Because it was apparently 'flexible,' or at least not tied to discretely
measurable activities, it was used to adjust nurses' productivity expectations, in the figures used in the staffing formula.

21 The formula is: workload index/$Y \times X$ (time) = staffing figure. For more
detailed discussion of the formula and how it was used to pass funding
cuts into nurse staffing, see Campbell (1984, esp. Chapter 4, 'Controlling the
Use of Nursing Labour,' 63–92).

22 'Indirect' care is a residual category – it might be time spent reading
instructions, time recording in the patient's record, or time for a nurse to
use the toilet.

23 Dorothy Smith's 'feminist sociology' (1987) details the social relations
embedded in women's (domestic, mothering) work that produce the conditions for men's achievements. She identified how, in the authorized sociological accounts about the world, men were organized to overlook the
conditions that allowed them to experience their work lives free from the
responsibility for managing mundane daily exigencies that held their work
together. We have identified the same system of social relations arising in
the everyday worlds of nurses.

24 So much so that the recommendations in a 1996 external nursing review at
the hospital where Rankin's research was conducted could comment
authoritatively on the workload measurement system in place at the hospital, the history of its use, and its potential for allocating (resources) more
effectively in that hospital. As well, the report noted the routine maintenance of a national database on patient classification and staffing information kept for comparison of staffing ratios among different hospitals.

25 Internal hospital decisions about the amount of budget to be allocated to
nursing labour would have reflected earlier decisions made at the ministry
level, e.g., the 1981 Ontario decision to stop reimbursing hospital cost over-
runs.

26 Patient classification continues to be an important part of the nursing management repertoire but is used less for scheduling staff than it was in the
beginning. By the end of the 1980s, patient classification had become

important in costing out nursing, to support nursing departments' claims for their share of funding allocated to hospitals on the basis of case-mix groupings (Mehmert et al. 1989).

2 'Three in a Bed'

1 Called 'chaotic' by the Steering Committee of the Western Canada Waiting List Project (Gordon Arnett, David Hadorn, and Steering Cte 2003) who have reported their early efforts to develop priority criteria for surgeons to help make assessments of prospective patients more objective and rational, thus fair. Physicians play the dominant role in managing waiting lists, and reliance on their judgement in this as in other clinical matters complicates rational management efforts.

2 Length of stay is planned prior to admission. Patients are informed about how long they will stay in the hospital and are expected to make arrangements for going home at the allocated standardized discharge time. (At this research hospital, patients are asked to sign a pre-admission agreement that commits them to making whatever arrangements required at home so that they can be discharged on time. Patients are advised that their surgery may be cancelled if they fail to comply. The standard discharge time is developed based on analysis of data from peer hospitals for similar surgeries.)

3 Alternate level of care (ALC) provides a means for screening patients related to whether the care provided *could* have been provided in an 'alternative' as opposed to 'hospital' setting. ALC is discussed in more detail in Chapter 3.

4 See Mykhalovskiy (2001) for a more detailed discussion about how physicians' and surgeons' resistance to reforming their approaches to care is being managed through discursive practices of health services research.

5 Health services research is a highly applied multidisciplinary field of research that addresses the structure, process, delivery and organization of health services (Mykhalovskiy 2001). It relies on quantitative and positivist research methods using complex statistical analysis to establish relationships between health services rendered and health outcomes for a broad selection of populations and services.

6 In the spring of 1997, Management Information Guidelines (MIS) guidelines were developed by the CIHI that established 'national standards that provide an integrated approach to managing financial and statistical data related to the operations of Canadian health service organizations' (Kerr et al. 1999: 255). The national standards are expected to inform decisions for 'planning and budgeting purposes, especially when projecting the impact

of expanding or downsizing of health service operations' (1999: 259). Key categories in the MIS statistical system include 'functional centre' (a category that monitors and calculates the accumulated costs of each hospital department such as health records, pharmacy, laboratory work, and nursing) and 'service recipient' (a category that relates costs of 'patient visits' to each hospital department). It is this system that contributes to 'case costing' predictions – aggregate calculations that report 'typical' costs for various procedures. For example, an Ontario case-costing initiative compared the average cost of coronary artery bypass graft (CABG) across four hospitals: University Health Network, London Health Sciences Centre, St Michaels Hospital, and Trillium Health Centre) (Couch and Sutherland 2004). The ADT system produces a great deal of the data entered into the categories of the MIS system.

7 See also Willis (2004) for an analysis of similar effects in Australian health care.

3 Doing the Right Thing at the Right Time

1 The social organization of the work of nursing's new front-line nurse leaders is examined in more detail in Chapter 4.

2 During the course of this research, the community hospital where Rankin first noticed ALC being used instituted major restructuring. Responding to trends in their ALC data, twenty acute care beds were closed on a medical wing of the hospital. Minor renovations were made, and these same beds were reopened as long-term-care beds. All the nursing staff in the adult medical and surgical units were given layoff notice. A reduction of the complement of registered nurses (RNs) and licensed practical nurses (LPNs) was achieved as the twenty 'new' long-term-care beds were staffed predominantly by less qualified long-term-care aides. New work rotations were developed, and the RNs and LPNs were required to reapply for fewer jobs under the jurisdiction of the British Columbia Health Labour Relations Act.

4 Managing Resistance to Restructuring

1 Their own presentation of 'the problem' – when they say 'threatening and inflammatory' – suggest as much.

2 A bed status report is a hospital-wide document which is faxed to each ward at 7:30 each morning. The report details how many patients are admitted and waiting in emergency for an available bed, how many 'same-day admit' surgical patients will be requiring a bed, and the number of

patient discharges that are required in order to accommodate incoming patients. Bed status reports are most commonly reported as 'negative' numbers of beds. One team leader interviewed described the bed status report as her way of knowing 'how hot the hospital is.'

3 Definition: *Acopia* the abnormal absence of 'coping.' This is a play on medical terminology using the common Latin prefix 'a-' meaning 'without' and the suffix '-ia' indicating an 'abnormal state.'

4 This competitive milieu is generated within a model that purports to value teams and 'teamwork,' while at the same time it pits one department against another to 'haggle over' patients who are deemed inappropriate candidates for hospital care.

5 In Chapter 6 we develop a more detailed account about how words from the nursing discourse are commandeered to develop nurses' changed organizational consciousness. We identify a 'double-sided' use of language that is professionally sanctioned.

5 Patient Satisfaction and the Management of Quality

1 Janet and her family members found that they had to get to the hospital very early in the morning, before breakfast, in order to get any information about Hannah's condition. The neurosurgeon who was overseeing Hannah's care regularly completed his rounds at this time of the day.

2 Throughout our description of Hannah's hospitalization we refer only to The Hospital in order to protect the anonymity of those people directly implicated by this research.

3 George Smith cites Hofstadter (1979) when he discusses the idea of recursivity and uses the term 'nested' to talk about this phenomenon of social relations. Smith uses an example of 'Russian dolls inside of Russian dolls' to emphasize how 'a story inside a story ... is part of a larger story and therefore has something of the same form' (1995: 33).

4 The *Vancouver Coastal Health Authority Newsletter* (2004) announces that CCHSA accreditation review is under way during 2003–5, 'an opportunity to evaluate the quality of care and services provided and compare VCH performance against national standards of quality.

5 The Agenda for Change, initiated by the (U.S.) Joint Commission on Accreditation of Healthcare Organizations in 1987, was a multiyear project that refocused accreditation actions towards improving quality by incorporating total quality management and continuous improvement and abandoning the term and the activities associated with 'quality assurance' (Rocchiccioli and Tilbury 1998: 244).

6 Re the elusive concept of quality, Carolyn L. Weiner (2004) asks if in our zeal for measuring it, 'we are measuring what is important [to health care] or simply making important what we can measure' (2004: 82).

7 A 'how-to' text approved by quality management guru, W. Edward Deming, who contributed a foreword.

8 This relationship between quality of care, the patient, and efficiency or reduction of waste can also be seen in messages from the Vancouver Coastal Health (VCH 2003) such as *Protecting Service Levels by Capturing Savings, Special Bulletin No. 30*, 16 Sept. 2003, that announced 'redesign strategies and new initiatives that will deliver $76.5 million in savings' so that service levels and quality of care can be maintained to patients, clients, and residents. In a follow-up announcement of initiatives undertaken, staff members were challenged to find creative ways of saving: 'If every staff member were able to save $20 per week for the rest of the fiscal year, we could save $10 million' (VCH Special Bulletin No. 32, 20 Oct. 2003).

9 Thus, patient satisfaction might be constructed in relation to human relations in the industrial relations discourse or to the caring discourses of nursing. For example, Sandra Haegert writes about patient satisfaction and nurses' caring explaining how 'caring also conveys the alleviation of vulnerability and the enabling of satisfaction ... [patients] being satisfied with nurses' caring lay in the principles of caring and the ethics of self' (2004: 436). In this example 'patient satisfaction' bears the conceptual imprints of 'a caring ethic' and 'authentic presencing' (2004: 436–7). Both concepts are fully entrenched in the nursing caring discourse.

10 Fuller and Smith (1991: 2) discuss evolving strategies to manage interactive service workers using customer feedback, strategies that require workers to 'read' the customer and to judge whether to be more 'friendly, speedy, flirtatious, solicitous or deferent.'

11 See Acorn and Barnett (1999) for a discussion of reliability and validity of patient satisfaction survey instruments. Our discussion of ideological practice addresses an entirely different level of trouble with social science methodology; (see also 'The Ideological Practice of Sociology,' Smith 1990a).

12 The Brief Summary of the 1998 patient and family survey claimed, as the final and apparently redeeming usefulness of the survey that otherwise offered a mixture of good and bad news, that it provided indicators for quality improvement.

13 Statistics Canada in association with Canadian Institute of Health Information and Health Canada conduct surveys, including three items on patient satisfaction with hospital care (StatsCan website)

14 The VCH Sustainable Development Update (Dec. 2003: 5) announced a number of educational sessions on 'change' for its managers.

15 Shelley Briggs (1998) identifies the extra difficulties faced by 'casual' nurses, including getting to know a new setting and its typical practices, both of which consume extra time and attention.

16 Smith also contrasts organizational accounts with scientific accounts. In the world of science, findings are contested, must be replicated, and so on. No such critical attention is given to organizational accounts. Just the opposite is true – organizational documents are carefully guarded from external scrutiny.

6 Language and the Reorganization of Nurses' Consciousness

1 Chapter 4 relates the activities of this group of activist nurses calling themselves Nurses United for Change (NUC), who reported critical incidents and eventually met with nursing consultants, who were conducting a review of nursing at their hospital. They related their experiences including what they saw as deterioration of the quality of care.

2 Smith cites not only Mead, but Vološ inov (1973), as she makes these arguments.

3 Workman (1996: 12) reports that Paul Martin, then federal finance minister, stated in his 1995 budget address that 'the last thing Canadians need is another lecture on the danger of the deficit.' By 1995 Martin could safely assume that widely held beliefs about a debt crisis made restraint measures infinitely reasonable to most Canadians.

4 Balbir Sandhu, RN, PhD, is a quality assurance counsellor at a hospital in Quebec. André Duquette, RN, PhD, and Suzanne Kérouac, RN, MN, MSc, are both associate professors at the Université de Montréal.

5 The articles selected for analysis here are not meant to be representative of any population or collection. Rather, we treat them as exhibits. Demonstrated in our analysis is the use of language that produces particular readings. We are interested in identifying that phenomenon. We make no claims about its prevalence. Readers can check for themselves how widespread these practices are in the nursing literature.

6 This heading quotes a 'layout banner' in the Canadian Nurse's presentation of the article by Fowlie, Francis, and Russell (2000: 30) that we analyse.

7 As Rankin discovered, the redesignation of shoulder surgery – rotator cuff repair – into the ambulatory care program (see Chapter 2) provided an instance of how more and more surgeries are treated as ambulatory care

procedures. In contemporary hospitals, 'day-surgeries' represent the largest proportion of surgical procedures being performed (CIHI 2004).

8 This heading is the title of the article by Wright and Leahey (1999) that is analysed here.

Conclusion

1 A hospital executive director interviewed by Rankin enthusiastically described his hospital's move to an organizational structure known as 'Integrated Programs.' As he described the changes his comment was: 'This move is really not going to impact nursing.'

2 Carolyn Weiner's (2000 and 2004) excellent research also recognizes this in what she calls the difference between rhetoric and reality.

3 A Canadian Nurses Association Report released in 2002 predicts a severe nursing shortage by the year 2011. 'The shortage is due to heavy workloads that are driving nurses into early retirement, and insufficient seats in nursing programs to meet expected demand. In addition, 21% of graduates from the years 1990 to 2000 are not practising in the profession – or not practising in Canada ... that's because they look at the work environment and the increasing workload and say "I can't do this" and they just quit' (Fletcher 2002: 15).

4 Two examples are Kaushal, Shojania, and Bates (2003) and Gawande and Bates (2000).

5 For instance, Dawn Pethybridge's (2004) Master's of Nursing thesis offers a contemporary look into the unrecognized work of nurses in an intensive care unit. What is recorded and attended to is that which supports physicians' treatment decisions. She makes a strong case for the relevance to good, ethical care of acting on local nursing knowledge, too.

6 In response to negotiations between provinces, territories, and the federal government on new funding for health care in the fall of 2004.

7 The reason cited by one hospital for contracting out 1,000 surgeries is its lack of sufficient surgical nurses.

References

Acorn, S., and J. Barnett. 1999. Patient satisfaction: Issues in measurement. *Canadian Nurse* 95(6): 33–6.

Al-Assef, A.F., and June Schmele, eds. 1993. *The textbook of total quality in health-care*. Delray Beach, Fla: St Lucie Press.

Annis Hammond, Sue. 1998. *The thin book of appreciative inquiry*. 2nd ed. Plano, Texas: Thin Book Publishing Co. http://www.thinbook.com.

Armstrong, Pat, Jacqueline Choiniere, Gina Feldberg, and Jerry White. 1994. *Take care: Warning signals for Canada's health system*. Toronto: Garamond Press.

Armstrong, Pat, Hugh Armstrong, Ivy Bourgeault, Jacqueline Choiniere, Eric Mykhalovskiy, and Jerry White. 2000. *'Heal thyself': Managing health care reform*. Aurora, Ont.: Garamond Press.

Arnett, Gordon, David Hadorn, and the Steering Committee of the Western Canada Waiting List Project. 2003. Developing priority criteria for hip and knee replacements: Results from the western Canada waiting list project. *Canadian Journal of Surgery* 46(4): 290–4.

Bakhtin, Mikhail M. 1981. *The dialogic imagination: Four essays*. Austin: University of Texas Press.

– 1986. *Speech genres and other late essays*. Trans. Vern. W. McGee. Caryl Emerson and Michael Holquist. Austin: University of Texas Press.

Bauman, Zygmunt. 2003. *Wasted lives: Modernity and its outcasts*. Cambridge: Polity Press.

Beardwood, Barbara, Vivienne Walters, John Eyles, and Susan French. 1999. Complaints against nurses: A reflection of 'the new managerialism' and consumerism in health care? *Social Science and Medicine* 48: 363–74.

Bennett, J., and J. Krasney. 1977. Health care in Canada. *The Financial Post*. Reprint of a series that appeared 26 March–7 May.

Block, Sheila. 2004. What does the increased federal funding for health care mean for Medicare advocates? *Behind the numbers: Economic facts, figures and analysis* 6(5):1–6. Canadian Centre for Policy Alternatives, Ottawa, 25 Oct.

Blum, B., ed. 1986. *Clinical information systems.* New York: Springer-Verlag.

Borins, Sandford. 2002. New public management, North American style. In *New public management: Current trends and future prospects,* ed. K. McLaughlin, S. Osborne, and E. Ferlie, 181–94. London: Routledge.

Bowker, Geoffrey, and Susan Leigh Starr. 1999. *Sorting things out: Classification and its consequences.* Cambridge: MIT Press.

Branowicki, Patricia A., and Herminia Shermont. 1997. Maximizing resources: A microanalysis assessment tool. *Nursing Management* 28(5): 65–70.

Briggs, Shelley. 1999. *The experience of 'casuals' working in critical care: Nurses talk about their work.* Master's of Nursing thesis. Faculty of Human and Social Development, University of Victoria.

British Columbia. 1991. *Closer to home: Summary of the Report of the British Columbia Royal Commission on Health Care and Costs.* Victoria: Author

Broadbent, Jane, and Richard Laughlin. 2002. Public service professionals and the new public management: Control of the professions in the public service. In *New public management: Current trends and future prospects,* ed. K. McLaughlin, S. Osborne, and E. Ferlie, 95–108. London: Routledge.

Burke, Ronald J., and Esther R. Greenglass. 2000. Hospital restructuring and downsizing in Canada: Are less experienced nurses at risk? *Psychological Reports* 87:1013–21.

CAEP (Canadian Association of Emergency Physicians). 2001. Submission to the commission on health care in Canada. *Emergency Medicine: Change and Challenge.* Section C – The case for national standards for hospital emergency services. Accessed Sept. 2004. http://www.caep.ca/002.policies/002-04.romanow/romanow-07.htm.

Campbell, Marie L. 1984. Information systems and management of hospital nursing: A study in the social organization of knowledge. PhD dissertation, Ontario Institute for Studies in Education (OISE), University of Toronto.

– 1988a. Management as ruling: A class phenomenon in nursing. *Studies in Political Economy* 27: 29–51.

– 1988b. Accounting for care: A framework for analyzing change in Canadian nursing. *Political issues in nursing: Past, present and future* 3: 45–69.

– 2001. Textual accounts, ruling action: The intersection of knowledge and power in the routine conduct of community nursing work. *Studies in Cultures, Organizations and Societies* 7(2): 231–50.

– 1992. Nurses' professionalism in Canada: A labour process analysis. *International Journal of Health Services* 22 (4):751–65.

– 1994. The structure of stress in nurses' work. In *Health illness and health care in*

Canada, ed. B. Singh Bolaria and Harley D. Dickinson, 592–608. 2nd ed. Toronto: Harcourt Brace and Co.

– 1995. Teaching accountability: What counts in nursing education? In *Knowledge, experience, and ruling relations: Studies in the social organization of knowledge*, ed. M. Campbell and A. Manicom, 221–33. Toronto: University of Toronto Press.

– 1998. Institutional ethnography and experience as data. *Qualitative Sociology* 21(1): 55–73.

– 2000. Knowledge, gendered subjectivity, and the restructuring of health care: The case of the disappearing nurse. In *Restructuring caring labour: Discourse, state practice and everyday life*, Sheila M. Neysmith, ed., 187–208. Don Mills: Oxford University Press.

Campbell, Marie L., and Nancy S. Jackson. 1992. Learning to nurse: Plans, accounts, and action. *Qualitative Health Research* 2(4): 475–96.

Campbell, Marie L., and Ann Manicom. 1995. *Knowledge, experience and ruling relations: Studies in the social organization of knowledge*. Toronto: University of Toronto Press.

Campbell, Marie, and Frances Gregor. 2002. *Mapping social relations: A primer in doing institutional ethnography*. Aurora, Ont.: Garamond Press.

Canada, Committee on the Costs of Health Services. 1970. *Task force reports on the cost of health services in Canada*, vol. 1. Ottawa: Author.

– National Health and Welfare. 1973. *Report of the Working Party on Patient Classification to the Advisory Committee on Hospital Insurance and Diagnostic Services*. Ottawa: Author.

Canadian Healthcare Association (CHA). 2004. Analysis of the 2004 health care plan. Accessed Nov. 2004. http://www.cha.ca/documents/ 2004HealthPlanAnalysisE.pdf.

CCHSA (Canadian Council on Hospital Services Accreditation). 2003. Accreditation recognition guidelines. *CCHSA survey guidelines*. Accessed Nov. 2004. http://www.cchsa.ca/pdf/survey_guidelines.pdf.

– 2004. Accreditation. Accessed Aug. 2004. http://www.cchsa.ca/ default.aspx?section=accrediitation&group=2.

CHSRF (Canadian Health Services Research Foundation). 1999a. *Annual Report*. Ottawa. Author.

– 1999b. Performance indicators, health services research and *Maclean's*. *Quid Novi: Newsletter of the Canadian Health Services Research Foundation* 2(4): 1, 5.

– 2000. Canada-wide healthcare report released. *Quid Novi: Newsletter of the Canadian Health Services Research Foundation* 3(2): 6.

– 2001. (banner) *Links: Newsletter of the Canadian Health Services Research Foundation* 4(1): 1.

CIHI (Canadian Institute of Health Information). 1997. *Understanding alternate level of care: Bulletin.* 28 May. Distributed by B.C. acute care facilities and the B.C. Ministry of Health.

– 2004. *National ambulatory care reporting system (NACRS).* Accessed Nov. 2004). http://secure.cihi.ca/cihiweb/disPage.jsp?cw_page=services_nacrs_e.

CIHR (Canadian Institutes for Health Research). 2000–1. *Annual Report.* Ottawa Author.

CNA (Canadian Nurses Association Fact Sheet Two). 1993. *Patient-Centred Care: High Quality; Lower Cost.* Ottawa: Author, June, 2 pages.

CNA (Canadian Nurses Association). 2002. *Code of Ethics for Registered Nurses.* Ottawa: Author.

Chua, W.F. 1991. The social manufacture of hospital product costs. Paper presented at the 3rd International Perspectives on Accounting Conference, University of Manchester, 8–10 July.

Couch, David, and Joan Sutherland. 2004. *OCCI Current and Future.* Ontario Ministry of Health. Accessed March 2005. http://www.healthinformation.on.ca/symp2004/presentations/Ontario %20Case% 20Cost%20Database_Couch_Sutherland.ppt.

Curran, C., and C. Gassert, 1998. Information management in a changing nursing environment. In *Clinical leadership in nursing,* ed. J. Rocchiccioli and M. Tilbury. Philadelphia: W.B. Saunders.

Dawson, Sandra, and Charlotte Dargie. 2002. New public management: A discussion with special reference to U.K. health. In *New public management: Current trends and future prospects,* ed. K. McLaughlin, S. Osborne, and E. Ferlie, 34–56. London: Routledge.

Dick, Jan, and Sharon Bruce. 1994. Cost containment: Doing more with less. In *Nursing management in Canada,* ed. Judith Hibberd and Mavis Kyle, 91–107. Toronto: Saunders.

Dickenson, Harley, D. 1996. Health reforms, empowerment and the democratization of society. In *Efficiency versus equality: Health reform in Canada,* ed. Michael Stingl and D. Wilson, 179–9. Halifax: Fernwood.

Ekstedt, Mirjam, and Ingegerd Fagerberg. 2005 Lived experiences of the time preceding burnout. *Journal of Advanced Nursing* 49(1): 59–68.

Equipe de Recherche Operationnelle en Santé. 1978. *PRN 76: An information system for nursing management.* Dept. d'Administration de la Santé, Université de Montréal.

Estabrooks, Carol. 1998. Will evidence-based nursing practice make practice perfect? *Canadian Journal of Nursing Research* 30(1): 15–36.

Evans, Robert G. 1984. *Strained mercy: The economics of Canadian health care.* Toronto: Butterworths.

Ferguson, J. 1994. *The anti-politics machine: 'Development,' depoliticization, and bureaucratic power in Lesotho.* Minneapolis: University of Minnesota Press.

Fletcher, Marla. 2002. Nursing by the numbers. *Canadian Nurse* 98(8): 14–16.

Fowlie, Pauline, Heather Francis, and Sunny Russell. 2000. A perioperative communication link with families. *Canadian Nurse* 96(6): 30–3.

Fuller, Colleen. 1998. *Caring for profit.* Vancouver: New Star Books.

Fuller, Linda, and Vicki Smith. 1991. Consumers' reports: Managing by customers in a changing economy. *Work, Employment and Society* 5(1): 1–16

Gallagher, P. 2004. How the metaphor of a gap between theory and practice has influenced nursing education. *Nurse Education Today* 24(4): 263–8.

Gallhofer, S., and J. Haslam. 1991. The aura of accounting in the context of a crisis: Germany and the First World War. *Accounting, Organizations, and Society* 4(2): 239–74.

Gawande, A.A., and D.W. Bates. 2000. The use of information technology in improving medical performance, part I. Information systems for medical transactions. *Medscape General Medicine e-journal* 2(1): E14.

Gerteis, Margaret, Susan Edgman-Levitan, Jennifer Daley, Jennifer Delbanco, and Thomas L. Delbanco. 1993. *Through the patient's eyes: Understanding and promoting patient-centred care.* San Francisco: Jossey-Bass.

Gervase, Bushe R. 2001. *Clear leadership.* Palo Alto, Ca.: Davies-Black.

Giovannetti, Phyllis, J.W. Mainguy, K.M. Smith, and L.V. Truitt. 1970. *The reliability and validity testing of a subjective patient classification system.* Vancouver, BC: Vancouver General Hospital.

Giovannetti, Phyllis, and Laverne McKague. 1973. *Patient classification system and staffing by workload index.* Saskatoon, Sask.: Hospital Systems Study Group.

Goar, L. 2004. Doctor's orders: Grain of salt. *The Toronto Star*, 13 August, A22.

Green, Carolyn J. 2004. The actualities of regional health board work: Implications for decision support design. PhD dissertation, School of Health Information Science, University of Victoria.

Hacking, Ian. 1990. *The taming of chance.* Cambridge: Cambridge University Press.

Haegert, Sandra. 2004. The ethics of self. *Nursing Ethics* 11(5): 434–44.

Harriss, Anne. 2004. Bridging the gap. *Occupational health* 56(6): 25–7.

Haylor, Martha. 2000. Clinical decision making model: A working paper. Presented at the Collaborative Nursing Program Conference, 20 April.

Haynes, R. Brian, Robert Hayward, and Jonathan Lomas. 1995. Bridges between health care research evidence and clinical practice. *Journal of the American Medical Informatics Association* 2(6): 342–50.

Health Services Redesign Plan, Vancouver Island Health Authority. 2003–6.

Accessed November 2004. http://www.viha.ca/pdf/mandate_page/
health_services_redesign_plan _03_06.pdf.

Henderson, Virginia. 1966. *The nature of nursing: A definition and its implications for practice, research and education.* New York: Macmillan.

Hibberd, J. M., and D.L. Smith. 1999. *Nursing management in Canada.* 2nd ed. Toronto: W.B. Saunders.

Hofstadter, Douglas, 1979. *Gödel, Escher, Bach: An eternal golden braid.* New York: Basic Books.

Ilcan, Suzan, and Lynne Phillips. 2003. Making food count: Expert knowledge and global technologies of government. *Canadian Review of Sociology and Anthropology* 40(4): 441–61.

– 2005. Circulations of insecurity: Globalizing food standards in historical perspective. In *Agricultural standards: The shape of the global food system.* Ed. Jim Bingen and Lawrence Busch, 51–72. Dordrecht: Kluwer Press.

Ingersoll, G.L. 2000. Evidence-based nursing: What it is and what it isn't. *Nursing Outlook* 48(4): 151–2.

Irvine, John, Ian Miles, and Jeff Evans, eds. 1979. *Demystifying social statistics.* London: Pluto Press.

ISO. 2004. ISO 9000 and ISO 14000 in plain language. Accessed Oct. 2004. http://www.1so.org/en/1s09000-14000/basics/general/basics_4.html.

Jackson, N.S. 2005. Adult literacy policy: Mind the gap. In *International handbook of educational policy,* ed. N. Bascia, A. Cumming, A. Datnow, K. Leithwood, and D. Livingston. Dordrecht: Springer.

Jelly-Shapiro, Joshua. 2004. Wasted lives. *Tikkun: A Bimonthly Jewish and Interfaith Critique of Politics, Culture and Society* 19(4): 72–4.

Joiner, Brian, L., in collaboration with Sue Reynard. 1994. *Fourth generation management: The new business consciousness.* New York: McGraw-Hill.

Kaushal R., K.G. Shojania, and D.W. Bates. 2003. Effects of computerized physician order entry and clinical decision support systems on medication safety: A systematic review. *Archives of Internal Medicine* 23(12): 1409–16.

Kerr, Christine, Colin Glass, Gillian McCallion, and Donald McKillop. 1999. Best-practice measures of resource utilization for hospitals: A useful complement in performance assessment. *Public Administration* 77(3): 639–50.

King, Imogene M. 1981 *A theory for nursing: Systems, concepts, process.* New York: Wiley.

Kirby, Michael J.L. 2002. *The health of Canadians: The federal role, final report.* Ottawa: Standing Senate Committee on Social Affairs, Science and Technology.

Kramer, Marlene.1974. *Reality shock: Why nurses leave nursing.* St Louis: Mosby.

– 1981. Why does reality shock continue? In *Current issues in nursing*, ed. J.C. McCloskey and H.K. Grace, 644–53. Boston: Blackwell Scientific.

Krawczyk, Marianne. 1989. Is MIS investment the key to solid hospital management? *Health Care*, June, 10–11.

Laffel, Glenn, and David Blumenthal. 1993. The case for using industrial quality management science in health care organizations. In *The textbook of total quality in healthcare*, ed. A.F. Al-Assaf and J. Schmele, 40–50. Delray Beach, Fla.: St Lucie Press.

Marx, Karl, and Frederick Engels 1970. *The German ideology*. New York: International Publishers.

MacDonnell, J.A.E. 1968. *Timing studies of nursing care in relation to categories of hospital patients*. Winnipeg: Deer Lodge Hospital.

Maclean's. 1999. The first ranking health report, 7 June. 112–23.

McCoy, Liza. 1998. Producing 'What the deans know': Cost accounting and the restructuring of post-secondary education. *Human Studies* 21: 395–418.

– 1999. Accounting, discourse and textual practices of ruling: A study of institutional transformation and restructuring in higher education. PhD dissertation. OISE, University of Toronto.

McLaughlin, Kate, Stephen Osborne, and Ewan Ferlie, eds. 2002. *New public management: Current trends and future prospects*. London: Routledge.

Mead, George Herbert. 1947. *Mind, self and society: From the perspective of a social behaviorist*. Ed. Charles W. Morris. Chicago: University of Chicago Press.

– 1992. *The individual and the social self: Unpublished work of George Herbert Mead*, ed. David L. Miller. Chicago: University of Chicago Press.

Mehmert, Peg, Carol Dickel, and Rosemary McKeighen. 1989. Computerizing nursing diagnosis. *Nursing Management* 20(7): 24–30.

Mykhalovskiy, Eric. 2001. On the uses of health services research: Troubled hearts, care pathways and hospital restructuring. *Studies in Cultures, Organizations and Societies* 7(2): 269–96.

Mykhalovskiy, Eric, and Lorna Weir. 2004. The problem of evidence-based medicine: Directions for social science. *Social Science and Medicine* 59: 1059–69.

NDP newswire, 25 Oct. 2004. Internal hospital e-mail alert puts lie to inflated health satisfaction numbers, says James. Accessed Oct. 2004. http://nid-876.newsdetail.bc.ndp.ca/upload/20041025133828_04125VIHA_email.pdf.

Ng, Roxana. 1995. Multiculturalism as ideology: A textual analysis. In *Knowledge, experience, and ruling relations: Studies in the social organization of knowledge*, ed. M. Campbell and A. Manicom, 35–48. Toronto: University of Toronto Press.

Ontario Hospital Association (OHA). 1982. Unpublished survey, March. Toronto: Author.

Orem, Dorothea. 1979. *Concept formalization in nursing: Process and product.* Boston: Little Brown.

Osborne, David, and Peter Plastrik. 2000. The reinventor's handbook: Tools for transforming your government. San Francisco: Jossey-Bass.

Pence, Ellen. 2001. Safety for battered women in a textually mediated legal system. *Studies in Cultures, Organizations and Societies* 7(2): 199–229.

Pethybridge, Dawn. 2004. Whose life is it anyway? End of life decision making in the ICU. Master's of Nursing thesis, Faculty of Human and Social Development, University of Victoria.

Petri, Donna. 2005. Decision making for nursing practice. *Collaborative Academic Education in Nursing (CAEN) curriculum guide.* Victoria: CAEN.

Petrie, Paul. 2003. *Maintaining quality health care at west Coast General Hospital.* Consultant's report presented to Port Alberni Mayor and VIHA CEO. Accessed Oct. 2004. http://www.viha.ca/news/pdf/port_alberni_report_nov_03.pdf.

Phillips, Lynne, and Suzan Ilcan. 2003. A world free from hunger: Global imagination and governance in the age of scientific management. *Sociologia Ruralis* 43(4): 434–53.

Potter, Patricia Ann, and Griffin Perry. 1997. Glossary. *Canadian fundamentals of nursing,* ed. Janet Ross Kerr and Mary Kosco Sirotnik. Toronto: Mosby Year Book.

Rachlis, M. 2004. *Prescription for excellence: How innovation is saving Canada's health care system.* Toronto: Harper Collins.

Rankin, Janet, M. 2001. Texts in action: How nurses are doing the fiscal work of health care reform. *Studies in Cultures, Organizations and Societies* 7(2): 251–68.

– 2003. Patient satisfaction: Knowledge for ruling hospital reform: An institutional ethnography. *Nursing Inquiry* 10(1): 57–65.

– 2004. How nurses practise health care reform: An institutional ethnography. PhD dissertation, Faculty of Human and Social Development, University of Victoria.

Regional Hospital. 1997. *Financial management and operational assessment: Review team report.* Confidential document.

RNABC (Registered Nurses Association of British Columbia). 2003. *Standards for nursing practice in British Columbia.* Vancouver: Author.

– 1996a. *Patient care delivery systems: Implications for nursing practice.* Vancouver: Author.

– 1996b. *Patient care delivery systems: An evaluation framework.* Vancouver: Author.

Robbins, Stephen, P. 1984. *Management: Concepts and practices.* Englewood Cliffs, NJ: Prentice-Hall.

Robbins, Stephen and Nancy Langton. 2003. *Organizational behaviour: Concepts, controversies, applications,* 3rd ed. Don Mills: Pearson Educational.

Rocchiccioli, Judith, T., and Mary S. Tilbury. 1998. *Clinical leadership in nursing.* Philadelphia: W.B. Saunders.

Romanow, Roy. 2002. *Building on values: The future of health care in Canada. Final report of the Commission on the Future of Health Care in Canada.* Saskatoon: The Commission.

Roy, Sr. Callista, and Sharon L. Roberts. 1981. *Theory construction in nursing: An adaptation model.* Englewood Cliffs, NJ: Prentice-Hall.

Sandhu, Balbir, Andre K. Duquette, and Suzanne Kérouac. 1992. How assignment patterns drive our professional practice. *Canadian Journal of Nursing Administration* 5(3): 9–14.

Shanahan, Marion, Marni Brownell, M. Loyd, and Noralou Roos. 1993. A comparative study of the costliness of Manitoba hospitals. *Medical Care.* 37 (Suppl) JS101.

Shanahan, Marion, Brownell, Marni, and Roos, Noralou. 1999. The unintended impacts of downsizing. *Medical Care* 37 (suppl 6) JS123–JS134.

Short, Ronald R. 1998. Learning in relationship. San Francisco: Learning in action technologies. Accessed August 2004. http://www.learninginaction. com.

Sibbald, Barbara, 1999. RN = really neglected, angry nurses say. *Canadian Medical Association Journal* 160(10): 1490–1.

Sjoberg K., and P. Bicknell. 1968. *Patient classification study.* Saskatoon, Sask.: Hospital Systems Study Group.

Smith, Donna Lynn, Donna Armann-Hutton, Noela Inions, and Dennis Hutton. 1999. Accountability, standards and quality. In *Nursing management in Canada,* Judith M. Hibberd and Donna Lynn Smith, 369–92. 2nd ed. Toronto: W.B. Saunders Canada.

Smith, D.E. 2005. *Institutional ethnography: A sociology for people.* Lanham, Md: AltaMira Press.

Smith, Dorothy E. 1987. *The everyday world as problematic: A feminist sociology.* Toronto: University of Toronto Press.

– 1990a. *The conceptual practices of power: A feminist sociology of knowledge.* Boston: Northeastern University Press.

– 1990b. *Texts, facts, and femininity: Exploring the relations of ruling.* New York: Routledge.

– 1999. *Writing the social: Critique, theory, investigations.* Toronto: University of Toronto Press.

– 2001. Texts and the ontology of organizations and institutions. *Studies in Cultures, Organizations and Societies* 7(2): 159–98.

Smith, George. 1995. Accessing treatments: Managing the AIDS epidemic in Ontario. In *Knowledge, experience, and ruling relations: Studies in the social organization of knowledge*, ed. M. Campbell and A. Manicom, 18–34. Toronto: University of Toronto Press.

Statistics Canada. 2004. Canadian community health survey. Accessed Sept. 2004. http://stcwww.statcan.ca/english/sdds/3226.htm. Includes links to topics and data on patient satisfaction, e.g., http://cansim2.statcan.ca/egi-win/ensmcgi.exe?

Suchman, Lucy. 1993. Do categories have politics? The language/action perspective reconsidered. In *Proceedings of the Third European Conference on Computer-Supported Work*, ed. G. DeMichelis, C. Simone, and K. Schmidt, 1–14. Milan, 13–17, Sept.

Taylor, Malcolm G. 1978. *Health insurance and Canadian public policy: The seven decisions that created the Canadian health insurance system*. Montreal: McGill-Queen's University Press.

The Hospital. 1995. *In pursuit of quality: An assessment of the quality of care and quality of worklife at (The Hospital): Summary report.*

– 1998a. *Survey introductory letter.*

– 1998b. *Through the patient's eyes: Patient survey.*

Thomas, Paul G. 1996. Beyond the buzzwords: Coping with change in the public sector. *International Review of Administrative Sciences* 62: 5–29.

Timmermans, Stefan, and Marc Berg. 2003. *The gold standard: The challenge of evidence-based medicine and the standardization of health care*. Philadelphia: Temple University Press.

Utley-Smith, Queen. 2004. 5 competencies needed by new baccalaureate graduates. *Nursing Education Perspectives* 25(4): 166–71.

VCH News. 2004. *Vancouver Coastal Health Authority Newsletter.* Accessed Aug. 2004. http:www.vch/ca/newslinks/current. (Public access to this site now forbidden.)

VCH Sustainable Development update. Dec. 2003. Accessed Aug. 2004. http://www.vcha.net/main/home.asp.

VCH Special Bulletin No. 30. 16 Sept. 2003. Accessed Aug. 2004. http://www.vch.ca.

VCH Special Bulletin No. 32. 20 Oct. 2003. Vancouver Health Authority special news bulletin. Accessed Aug. 2004. http://wwwvcha.net/main/home.asp.

Vološ inov, V.I. 1973. *Marxism and the philosophy of language*. Trans. by I.R. Titunik. New York. Academic Press.

Weiner, Carolyn. 2000. *The elusive quest: Accountability in hospitals*. New York: Aldine de Gruyter.

– 2004. Holding American hospitals accountable: Rhetoric and reality. *Nursing Inquiry* 11(2): 82–90.

Weisinger, Hendrie. 1998. *Emotional intelligence at work*. San Francisco: Jossey-Bass.

Willis, Eileen. 2004. Accelerating control: An ethnographic account of the impact of micro-economic reform on the work of health professionals. PhD dissertation, Department of Social Inquiry, University of Adelaide.

Windle, Pamela E. 1994. Critical pathways: An integrated documentation tool. *Nursing Management* 25(9): 80F–80P.

Workman, Thom W. 1996. *Banking on deception: The discourse of fiscal crisis*. Halifax: Fernwood.

Woodward, C.A., H.S. Shannon, C. Cunningham, J. McIntosh, B. Lendrum, D. Rosenbloom, and J. Brown, 1999. The impact of re-engineering and other cost reduction strategies on the staff of a large teaching hospital: A longitudinal study. *Medical Care* 37(6): 556–69.

Wright, Lorraine, and Maureen Leahey. 1999. Maximizing time, minimizing suffering: The 15-minute (or less) family interview. *Journal of Family Nursing* 5(3): 259–75.

Yalnizyan, Armine. 2004. Paul Martin's permanent revolution. *Alternative Federal Budget 2004*. Technical paper No. 3. Ottawa: Canadian Centre for Policy Alternatives.

Yamamoto, Hiromi. 2003. New public management – Japan's practice. Institute for International Policy Studies. Accessed Aug. 2004). http://www.iips.org/bp293e.pdf.

Index

Accountability, 120, 181; built-in flaw of, 174; era of, 26; nursing restructured by, 22; people's expectations of, 174; as taught to nurses, 178; a textual product, 21, 98; used in a double-sided way, 172

Accounting logic (logic of accountability), 14–22, 66, 87, 185n7; and efficiency, 64; embedded in technology, 46; new public management and, 14, 132, 139–40, 164; nurses and, 75, 142, 168; in nursing discourse, 149; patient-centred care and, 124, 137; speech genre and, 144–5

Accreditation (of health care organizations), 123, 132, 193nn4–5

Actuality-data-theory circuit, 128, 135

Acute care (*see also* Bed): admissions to, 11, 45; discharge from, 84; in the home, 100; management of: bed occupancy, 25 (*see also* admission, discharge, and transfer system, 50–8); benchmarks for, 64; costs of, 77; inpatient days, 64

Administration, of health care, 11; textual realities of, 85; transformation of, 7

Administration (public), 11, 14. *See also* new public management

Administrative knowledge, trumps local judgment, 57

Admission, discharge, and transfer system (ADT), 50–8; account of beds occupied, 51; definition of, 20; numerically based monitoring, 50; organizes nurses' attention, 45; statistics amassed by, 55; technology of governance, 45; a textual reality, 20

Alternate level of care (ALC), 53, 66, 76–88, 102, 191n3; designation, 6; designation form 78; off index days 103

Alternative account, 175–80; making of, 22

Ambulatory care, 48, 55, 153; growth in, 153, 195–6n7; improves (bed) utilization, 64

Analysis (*see also* Institutional ethnography), 16–18, 173, 185n8; approach to, 17; in this book, 7; ethnographic, 64, 112; experiential